Chicken Soup for the Soul

Healthy Living:

*Back Pain*

# Chicken Soup for the Soul
## Healthy Living:
### *Back Pain*

Jack Canfield

Mark Victor Hansen

Jonathan Greer, M.D., FACP, FACR

**Health Communications, Inc.**
**Deerfield Beach, Florida**

*www.hcibooks.com*
*www.chickensoup.com*

We would like to acknowledge the many publishers and individuals who granted us permission to reprint the cited material.

*From Back Pain to Back Bends.* Reprinted by permission of Ingrid Bairstow. ©2006 Ingrid Bairstow.

*Regaining Life.* Reprinted by permission of Janice G. Bazen. ©2006 Janice G. Bazen.

*What I Am Made Of.* Reprinted by permission of Andi Blaustein. ©2006 Andi Blaustein.

*Smoke Free, Pain Free.* Reprinted by permission of Liz Clark. ©2006 Liz Clark.

*The Spirit Can't Be Broken.* Reprinted by permission of Mary Cook. ©2006 Mary Cook.

*(Continued on page 133)*

**Library of Congress Cataloging-in-Publication Data is available from the Library of Congress**

©2006 Jack Canfield and Mark Victor Hansen
ISBN 0-7573-0522-9

Publisher: Health Communications, Inc.
          3201 S.W. 15th Street
          Deerfield Beach, FL 33442–8190

*Cover design by Larissa Hise Henoch*
*Inside book design by Lawna Patterson Oldfield*
*Inside book formatting by Dawn Von Strolley Grove*

# Contents

# Introduction: You Can Beat Back Pain

Our spine keeps us upright, allows us to get around, and lets us twist and bend in a variety of positions. But we often take this amazing mechanism for granted—until something happens that makes us take notice.

Let's get the bad news out of the way: Most of us will, in our lifetime, experience back pain—and for a few us, it can be agonizing and debilitating. Back pain is the leading cause of disability and absenteeism within all industrialized nations. The good news is that most people recover and only a few are left with chronic complaints.

The source of back pain is usually obscure. Whenever we feel a twinge we say, "It's my disc" or "It's my sciatic nerve" or "It's my bone spur." But in reality, most of the time we can't really pinpoint where the pain comes from. This is why both the diagnosis and management of back pain can be such a challenge for health-care providers.

In my nineteen years of practice as a rheumatologist, I've seen back pain virtually every day. I've learned that not all back pain is the same and that people have their individual set of circumstances and experiences related to their pain. In some cases, their pain is a discomfort they ignore, in others the pain is serious and life threatening, and in still others the pain isn't from their back at all—though they think it is. I've also learned that no two patients with back pain can be treated the same way. Part of the art of medicine is understanding how a patient's pain is manifested and what therapies are most appropriate for them. Another part of the art of medicine is determining how and when to turn to medications and surgery, which requires the physician to weigh the patient's risk factors and the potential benefits.

In this book, we'll explore the various issues surrounding your back. The book will enhance your knowledge, clarify common misconceptions, help you to understand the possibilities you face and assist you in finding the best care. Being informed is being empowered—and you'll fare better when you understand your condition and cooperate with your doctor in the healing process.

—Jonathan M. Greer, M.D., FACP, FACR

## A Reason for the Pain

Everything happens for a reason. My mother must have told me this fifteen thousand times if she told me once. The frustrating part is she nearly always turned out to be right.

When I moved to southern Germany for work, I had no plans to learn the German word for herniated disc. But just a month into my teaching job in Heilbronn I'd added *Bandscheibenvorfall* to my meager vocabulary. And I'd learned how the tiniest false move could send waves of bone-grating pain from the base of my spine to every cell of my body. The pressure of the bulging disc on my spinal cord had me not just feeling pain, but hearing it in a kind of bodily shriek, tasting it as I tried not to scream and seeing it as my vertebrae freakishly contracted and my body twisted any way it hoped might alleviate the agony.

The crash course in the German medical system that followed gave me countless physiotherapy sessions and a regular regime of swimming, walking and faithful observance of the prescribed exercises.

A year later, I'd almost forgotten it had ever happened. And that was the problem.

No pain, no brain. I used to hear it the other way around, but this time the lack of any reminders made me stupid enough to think that taking care of my body had become less important. On New Year's Day, alone in my flat and with all my girlfriends still away on their Christmas holidays, I woke up unable to walk more than a few meters. Almost worse than the immobility was the fear that the horrifying original degree of pain would return.

I had a very casual date scheduled for the evening. An ex-student of mine and I had agreed to meet for a drink at a nearby pub. But no matter how nearby it was, there was no chance I could make it. I suggested we cancel our plans, and he offered to bring the drink around instead and keep me company. The evening saw me lying on the sofa trying to be a good host, with little success. A call came the next day: he'd found a doctor who was open over the New Year break and had managed to wrangle an appointment for me, something my still-shaky German could never have done. Did I need a lift?

Did I ever. After he brought me home from the doctor, he stayed to play cards, to have lunch, to have dinner . . . and he's barely left since. We're getting married next year. I religiously do my back exercises now, and swim and walk as much as possible. It's clear to me now why I had to suffer through this back pain, and I don't need it anymore. Now I need to be fit and healthy to enjoy the time with my dream man. I'm one of the lucky ones, whose back pain can be controlled and almost eliminated with the right exercises, so I'm taking advantage of it: but I'm still grateful for it. And once again, my mother was right.

♥ *Amanda Kendle*

# Where Does It Hurt?

Point at your pain. Go ahead . . . no one is looking.

If you pointed to your rear end, you might be in for a surprise. Most patients who think they have hip pain point to their posterior buttock, but in reality, this pain originates in the low back and is called *referred pain*. This sensation happens when signals from several areas of the body travel through the same nerve pathways on the way to the spinal cord and brain.

The point of that little pointing exercise is to show you that back pain isn't as simple as it may seem, and that pain in other parts of your body—such as in your hips or legs—may actually be a sign of back problems.

In later chapters you'll learn all about the different varieties of back woes and what you can do about them—but right now, you need to know how to describe your pain so the doctor can diagnose you properly and set you on the path to feeling great. Here are some questions to ask yourself; you may want to write the answers in the worksheet at the end of this chapter so that you can show them to your health-care provider.

## When did the pain start?

If you first felt the ouch when you lifted that heavy box at work, that's important information.

Or perhaps the pain came on gradually after you joined a bowling league, started a new job or went through an emotional rough patch. Also note what time of the day the pain is at its worst; wear-and-tear pain tends to gets worse as the day goes on, while inflammatory back pain is worse in the A.M. and improves with movement during the day.

### Where is the pain?

Try to pinpoint where you're hurting. Is it in your upper or lower back? Which side of your back hurts? Is the pain in your hip, and if so, which part of the hip? (Pain in the groin area is most likely from the hip joint; pain in the side of the hip may be bursitis; and pain in the buttock is usually from the back.) Or maybe it's your leg that hurts. You can even use a diagram of the human body to circle the areas that hurt. Another thing to consider is whether the pain stays in one place or radiates to other parts of the body.

### What is the pain like?

Words you can use to describe pain include *burning, throbbing, shooting, stinging, radiating, intermittent* (comes and goes), *sore* and *fluffy*—okay, maybe not fluffy.

### How does the pain affect you?

Let your doctor know how your back pain affects your life. For example, you may have trouble sitting at a desk at work, bending to pick up toys from the floor, reaching for a box of cereal on the top shelf at the supermarket, playing with your kids or participating in your favorite activity. Be sure to add whether the pain affects you at night, and whether you have numbness, weakness, or loss of bladder or bowel control, because these are all red flags.

## Does anything make the pain better or worse?

Perhaps lying in bed or using an ice pack eases the hurt, or sitting too long in one position makes the pain worse. Think about walking versus standing versus lying down, and note how each affects the pain.

## How much does it hurt?

It can help your doctor if you're able to rate your pain. You can use a range of words such as *no pain, a little pain* and *lots of pain,* or perhaps a scale from zero to ten, with zero being no pain at all and ten being the worst pain ever. Using a system like these to rate your pain helps your health-care provider determine what the problem is, prescribe a treatment, assess the effectiveness of the remedy and adjust the treatment when necessary.

## Keep a Pain Diary

No, we don't mean that you have to spill your deepest secrets in a flower-covered, locked diary. We mean that you should keep a log of your pain: when, where and how much your back hurts, what activities you took part in that day, what your mood was and anything else you think might be important. Keeping a pain diary may help you and your doctor see connections that you might have missed otherwise, such as that your pain occurs when you're feeling stressed or that it feels more intense when you sit too long at work. The diary can also help you track which medical treatments and lifestyle changes work best for you. So let's get started: "Dear Diary . . ."

## *Think about . . .*
## my treatment goals

The reasons I want to heal my back pain are:

__ To be able to participate in my favorite sport.

__ To be able to play with my kids—pain free.

__ To do a better job at work.

__ To allow me to be a better spouse.

__ To be able to sleep.

__ To function better in the home.

__ To enhance my sense of well-being.

__ To help other people, whether carrying groceries for my elderly neighbor or helping a friend move.

_____

_____

_____

## Think about . . .
### how it feels

This is where I can write the answers to my pain questions. I'll show this worksheet to my health-care provider.

When did the pain start?

_____

_____

_____

Where is the pain?

_____

_____

_____

What is the pain like?

_____

_____

_____

How does the pain affect me?

_____

_____

_____

Does anything make the pain better or worse?

_____

_____

_____

How much does my back hurt on a scale from zero to ten?

0   1   2   3   4   5   6   7   8   9   10

## Regaining Life

It was the end of 2002 and my life was in shambles. My marriage was over, I hugged my friends and family good-bye, and finally let go of any dreams that I would ever return to work. To say I was in the throes of major depression would be an understatement.

I had been living with back pain most of my adult life due to degenerative disc disease and arthritis. Bone grafts and rod placements were used to stabilize my spine in 2001, but four months later the pain returned. I couldn't leave home without my cane in hand and couldn't shop unless the store provided an electric handicap cart. I was sent to a pain management clinic that prescribed medications to help me function better. I never knew how far I was going to be able to walk before the pain would hit and stop me in my tracks. Many times I was left frozen in place while someone ran to get the car or a wheelchair.

With mounting medical bills and my income gone, I filed for bankruptcy. I gave up the house I loved and was so proud of. I used to spend hours gardening; I was reduced to staring out the window at the empty field dreaming of what I would plant if I could. Slowly, it seemed that everything that had ever brought me joy was gone. I couldn't go to the stadium and sit to watch my daughter play in the marching band or my sons play football because the hard benches hurt my back. I would pretend it didn't bother me to be left behind but there were many tears shed in silence.

It was just after moving back in with my mom that I had the worst night of pain in my life. I don't remember what I had been doing that day, only the gradual onset of breakthrough pain and going to bed to rest. I awoke not able to move or turn over without screaming in pain. My family called 911. I screamed as the medics moved me with a sheet to the gurney.

It took the medical personnel hours and much morphine to get my pain under enough control that I could move. I was discharged with orders to see a surgeon.

All of this led to another MRI and another surgery with rod placement and bone graft. I knew what was expected of me in rehab and that made the process easier. I found myself progressing much quicker than with the previous surgery.

I remember the day of my ultimate challenge. I

was on a table at physical therapy wearing my turtle-shell brace and working out with leg weights when another patient's wife approached me to talk. She told me she recognized the brace and we began to share the histories of our back surgeries as I continued to work out. I shared that my goal was to someday be able to return to work. She quickly said I would never be able to work again, that she hadn't and we had the same medical history. As she walked away I felt tears and anger of frustration. I thought to myself, *We may have the same histories but we don't have the same resolve!* I began to work even harder at my strengthening exercises.

Within three months I had easily weaned myself off all pain meds. I was walking farther and began leaving my cane behind. I pushed myself harder until I learned what my limits were going to be. I could soon walk more than a mile before feeling any discomfort and even that was tolerable. I felt like a new woman!

After nine months of freedom from pain pills, walkers and canes, I started interviewing for jobs. I knew it would take a special company to give me a chance to return to the work I loved and also be willing to work within my limitations: no lifting, twisting or bending, no standing or sitting for long periods and the ability to work at my own pace. On my second interview I was hired as a home health

RN, the same job I had left four years before. I was allowed to start slow, just a few patients a week, and when I tried to work a full-time schedule and back pain started to return, the company allowed me to slow down to a part-time pace I could handle.

I have been working for two years now and cannot express the joy I have of walking into a patient's home and saying . . .

"Never give up."

♥ *Janice Bazen*

# Ouch! Acute Back Pain

You're hoisting a heavy box when suddenly your lower back cries out, "I give up!" and the pain makes you head for the couch. Or maybe you slip on a patch of ice and end up staring at the sky with your back in agony. Or perhaps your lower back starts giving you grief for no known reason at all.

*Acute* pain is pain that lasts anywhere from a moment up to three to six months or pain that comes from tissue damage (such as when you slipped on that ice). It can be deep, aching, dull, burning or spasmodic, and can stay in one area of the back or travel down one or both legs.

Acute low back pain is the fifth most common reason for all physician visits, so you're certainly not alone! A few causes of acute low back pain include back strain, osteoarthritis (where cartilage in your joints breaks down so that bones rub against one another) and disc herniation (where a disc—the cushion between your vertebrae—moves out of place and presses against a nerve).

It's a good idea to get medical help for acute low back pain. The longer the pain lasts, the greater the chance of it developing into a chronic pain problem. You might also develop depression or anxiety, and you may avoid exercise to prevent making the pain worse—only to discover that lack of exercise leads to weight gain, obesity-related diseases and weaker back muscles!

Luckily, most acute low back pain is caused by something unscary, like a strained muscle, and is rarely a sign of a serious disease. But you should immediately see your health-care provider for treatment of acute low back pain if:

- You experience numbness or difficulty moving a leg. Such sensations can signal nerve damage, either to the spinal cord or to the nerve roots that travel from the spine down the legs.

- You're pregnant. Some women feel the pain in their back instead of the usual locations when they go into labor, especially when the baby is traveling through the birth canal face up instead of face down. This is called *back labor*.

- The pain is worse when you're lying still. Cancer is always a concern when rest pain is described.

- You have a fever, feel poorly and have severe symptoms such as a bad headache. Infection is a possibility here, specifically meningitis, disc infection or even bone infection.

- You're over 60. Older patients are more likely to have infections, nerve damage, cancer or compression fractures from osteoporosis.

- You have pain in your left arm or the chest. Such pain commonly signals a heart attack, so your physician will first want to rule out heart disease, then other causes, such as pneumonia, pulmonary embolism or muscle strain.

- You have loss of bladder or bowel control. This condition implies damage to the spinal nerves that control bladder and bowel function and requires immediate attention.

- You've been taking steroids for many years. Steroids cause the bones to become weak and brittle (osteoporosis), which can lead to collapsed vertebrae or compression fractures.

You'll probably want to see a physician even if you lack these symptoms or conditions—after all, back pain is no fun! Your doctor might refer you to a physical therapist or chiropractor (see page 81 for more information on these professionals), recommend an exercise regimen, prescribe medication or send you to a lab for a scan such as an MRI or a CT scan (see page 69 for the scoop on these and other tools health-care providers use to diagnose back pain). Acute disc herniation occurs in only 5 percent of acute back pain cases, and this pain usually responds well to time, exercise and medication. Very few people in this situation need surgery!

Don't try to exercise the pain away on your own; let a doctor recommend specific exercises for you, and peruse the following list of treatments that you can try at home:

- Take a nonsteroidal anti-inflammatory drug (NSAID), such as aspirin or ibuprofen. This will not only help relieve pain, but also reduce any inflammation in the back. Read and follow the label's instructions. Consult your health-care provider before taking an NSAID if you are on blood thinners or have a history of asthma, stomach ulcers or any health condition that could be worsened by such medication. Stop taking this drug if you experience stomach discomfort, swollen legs, rashes, elevated blood pressure or chest pain.

- Apply a cold pack to the painful area for 20 to 30 minutes, repeating every two hours as needed for up to 48 hours after the injury. After a day or two of the cold shoulder, so to speak, use heat treatment on the affected area: apply a heating pad to the painful area for 20 to 30 minutes, repeating every two hours as needed. Inspect your skin often to make sure your skin isn't being damaged by the extreme temperatures.

- Get a massage—a regular massage, mind you, not a deep-tissue pounding. Physical therapists and chiropractors both use massage, and these services are often covered by health insurance. Stop the massage, though, if you experience any of the "red flags" listed earlier.

- Stretch. Lie on your back with your knees bent. Grasp one knee with both hands and slowly pull it toward your chest. Hold the knee for a few seconds to get a gentle stretch, then release it. Repeat with the other leg.

- Lie on your back with a pillow under your knees to reduce traction on the sciatic nerve (the nerve that runs from the lower back down the back of each leg).

Acute pain gets better after a few weeks 95 percent of the time, so if your back is still hurting a month after the initial pain, see your health-care provider again.

## Give Yourself a Lift

Using an improper lifting technique when hoisting something heavy can hurt your back. Squat down instead of bending at the waist so that your legs do the lifting. Hold the object close to your body to keep the weight from pulling your torso forward and straining your back.

## Back Pain Myths

**Myth #1:** You should rest your back until it feels better.

Studies show that people who rest less and try to stay active feel better faster than those who languish in bed for days on end. Try to rest for no longer than 24 to 48 hours.

**Myth #2:** When you hurt your back, lie on the floor or a firm mattress.

The floor doesn't offer enough support for your aching back—and it's harder to get up from when you do want to move around. (Remember the "I've fallen and I can't get up" commercial? She was on the floor, not in bed!) If you need to lie down, choose the bed—preferably one with a soft or pillow-top mattress, as experts no longer recommend firm mattresses for back health.

Think about . . .
my opinions

The methods I'll use when I experience acute
back pain include:

\_\_ Taking a nonsteroidal anti-inflammatory
drug, such as aspirin or ibuprofen.

\_\_ Using an ice pack.

\_\_ Using a heating pad or taking a hot shower.

\_\_ Getting a massage.

\_\_ Stretching.

\_\_ Making an appointment with my doctor if
nothing else helps!

## Smoke Free, Pain Free

My back injury may have saved my life.

It all began in one of the worst years of my life. My dad had just died of heart problems, I lost my job and my husband took a new position that forced us to move thousands of miles away.

In the chaos of such big change, I ignored my health and started smoking cigarettes again. I'd started smoking years before in an attempt to stay awake during college test weeks. I'd started and stopped many times since, never feeling I was truly addicted.

Yet here I was, stealing increasingly long moments away from unpacking and sending out resumes. Some days, I went through half a pack, and on weekends, it would sometimes stretch to two. Long after the boxes were empty, I was still smoking more than I had before.

Winter set in. My husband hated the smell and wouldn't let me smoke in the house, so there I stood, puffing away outside in the chilly winds on our tiny wooden deck.

Then one night, cigarettes in hand, I stepped outside and—whooops! My feet slid across the ice-covered steps and into the air. I hit the deck with a bang, smashing my hip into the step.

My husband came running. He helped me up, but shook his head in disgust as I immediately lit my cigarette, still shaking from the fall. My lower back was in pain, but my need for tobacco was greater.

An enormous swollen bruise rose up on my hip. Weeks later, after it faded, the pain was still there. By then, I had found a new job, but my back was so sore that I could barely stay seated in the cushy chair. When my husband wanted to go out to eat, to celebrate a big deal he'd just closed, I had to beg off: it was just too painful to sit for an hour in a restaurant.

So I saw a doctor, then another, then another, all of whom couldn't quite figure out what was wrong. I tried physical therapy and acupuncture, massage and pain pills, and anything else I thought might help, until finally one day a doctor said, I know what this is: you've torn a ligament.

He prescribed a new kind of therapy, but warned me if it didn't work, he might have to operate. Then he asked me something none of the other doctors had asked: "Do you smoke?"

"Sometimes," I said. I didn't think it was his business: I never smoked in public, never carried the cigarettes in my purse. To me, smoking was something I did in private, on my deck. I wasn't sure why he was asking me about it.

"Then quit," he said.

"I've tried," I said. "Look, I don't smoke that much—just a few each day."

He gave me a stern look.

"Okay, sometimes I smoke more than that on weekends. But it's no big deal."

He sighed and sat down in the chair across from me. "Let me tell you something. I've been operating on people's backs for 30 years. Usually they're successful. Sometimes they're not. So a few years back, I started taking a closer look at the ones that didn't work."

*Oh no. A lecture,* I thought, squirming on the examining table.

"Guess what?" he said. "Almost every one of those patients smoked. So now I tell my patients, if you can't quit smoking, I'm going to have a tough time fixing your problems. You're working against me every time you pick up a cigarette."

I was surprised. I knew smoking caused a range of diseases. I told him I didn't see how it was connected to my back.

"We know smoking causes problems with the

respiratory system, and with circulation," he explained. "Maybe when you smoke, the ligaments and muscles of your back aren't getting the blood flow they need to heal. Maybe there's not as much oxygen in your blood. Who knows? I'm just telling you what I've seen, right here in this office."

I pondered this information. If smoking made it harder to recover from surgery, then what was it doing to my back injury right now?

"Promise me you'll think about it," he said, and I nodded.

That night, when I stepped out onto the deck for a cigarette, I didn't enjoy it very much. As the smoke curled upward, I began to associate it with the searing pain, all the agony and frustration my injury had brought into my life.

That week, I smoked my last cigarette. The new back therapy worked so well that within weeks my husband and I went to celebrate—with a long, romantic dinner in a candlelit restaurant.

Now, years later, my back pain is gone forever. And thanks to a very good doctor, it left me even healthier than before, free from the toxic effects of smoking.

♥ *Liz Clark*

# Doc, My Back Always Hurts: Chronic Back Pain

It's been three months since your back started hurting—and the pain just won't leave you alone. You may be suffering from chronic back pain, which is more common in people who:

- Smoke.
- Have had a past back injury or acute back pain. (See info on acute back pain.)
- Don't exercise.
- Are extremely tall.
- Are very overweight.
- Work in jobs that require heavy, repetitive lifting.
- Are often exposed to vibrations while riding in motor vehicles—especially tractor trailers—or industrial machinery.
- Participate regularly in certain sports such as cross-country skiing or soccer.
- Have poor posture.
- Are tall, overweight, smoking and playing competitive-lift soccer after slouching for hours in an 18-wheeler.

As you can see, the list is long and varied—but wait, there's more! Chronic back pain, which can originate in the bones, muscles or discs (the cushioning between the vertebrae), can also be caused by conditions such as osteoarthritis, fibromyalgia, car accidents and other problems. What's more, the type of pain can vary greatly, from tingling to stabbing, and can be mild or severe. With so many possible variations, finding the source of the pain can be difficult.

And sometimes, the problem that caused the back pain in the first place—such as an injury or medical condition—may be completely healed, but you still feel pain. (Feeling pain from a stimulus like touch that doesn't normally produce pain is called *allodynia*.)

So you can see how chronic back pain might be difficult to diagnose! But don't despair: read on to learn what to expect when you visit the doctor and what you can do to prevent or alleviate chronic back woes.

## Getting the Scoop on Your Back Pain

Your health-care provider needs to find out where the pain is coming from, so she'll compile a thorough history of your back problems and perform a physical examination. She may send you out for an X-ray, bone scan, computerized tomography (CAT scan) or magnetic resonance imaging (MRI) so that she can complement your history with a peek under the hood, as it were. (Flip to page 69 for information on the different types of diagnostic tools your doctor may use.)

If your doctor can't find anything physically wrong with you, she may suspect that the problem is psychological. No, that doesn't mean the pain is "all in your head"—it means that emotional factors such as stress and depression can cause chronic back pain.

## Getting Better

Unfortunately, the problems underlying chronic back pain can be hard to pinpoint. The good news is that there are a multitude of treatments aimed at reducing the pain and keeping you comfortable and active.

- **Prescription and Over-the-Counter (OTC) Drugs**

   Depending on your condition, your doctor may prescribe a medication such as a muscle relaxant or suggest you take an OTC nonsteroidal anti-inflammatory drug (NSAID). Check out page 98 for the details on medications.

- **Injections**

   Getting needled can relieve a bigger pain in your back. Your doctor may inject an anesthetic or a steroid (or both) into the affected areas to help put the kibosh on chronic back pain. Steroids reduce inflammation of the muscles or other tissues; inflammation can cause swelling, nerve irritation and spasms.

### • Alternative Therapies

Acupuncture (yep, more needles!), massage, hypnotherapy and meditation are some alternative therapies that can help relieve the ouch of chronic back pain. Check out page 107 for the details.

### • Physical Therapy or Chiropractic

Your doctor may refer you to a physical therapist or a chiropractor. Page 81 has the story on these professionals.

### • Exercise

Moving your body can help you develop a strong, flexible back that's less likely to give you grief. A good back-boosting exercise program includes aerobic exercise like dancing or walking, stretching, and strength training (especially exercises that focus on your stomach, back and leg muscles). Talk to your health-care provider before beginning a new exercise regimen, because going it alone may hurt more than it heals.

• **Therapy**

Back pain can affect your whole life, from your mood to how you interact with your family, and it can be a drag on every other activity. A trained pain specialist, psychologist or psychiatrist can help you develop skills to cope with the negative emotions that you may feel. (These emotions can also make your back pain worse; see the sidebar on page _____.)

• **Kicking Butts**

Smoking, on top of all its other health drawbacks, puts you at risk for degenerative disc disease, osteoporosis and arthritis, and it lowers the pain threshold so your back hurts more than it normally would. Ask your doctor for help kicking the habit; she may recommend support groups, helpful resources, or over-the-counter or prescription medications that make quitting easier.

• **Surgery**

Believe it or not, one of the surgical options for certain back problems is to implant a metal disc replacement in the spine. It's enough to make the Six Million Dollar Man jealous! Of course, surgery isn't something to be undertaken lightly, and very few patients would qualify for such treatment. (See page 89 for more details on the different types of surgery.)

## Chronic Back Pain
## Do's and Don'ts

DO quit smoking.

DON'T slouch, especially when sitting for long periods of time. A lumbar support cushion or footstool can help you sit upright, so feel free to pester your boss for this essential health supplement.

DO lose excess weight—and keep it off. (See page 119 for more info.)

DON'T do exercises that strain the back, such as sit-ups with your legs straight or leg lifts performed while lying on your back.

## ⚕ *Think about . . .*
## my health history

Here's information that can help my health-care provider diagnose and treat my back pain.

My previous back injuries: _____

_____

My previous back surgeries: _____

_____

Any other medical conditions: _____

_____

Any family history of back pain: _____

_____

Medications I'm taking now for any condition:

_____

My history of depression or anxiety: _____

_____

Stressors in my life: _____

_____

My job requirements (including sitting for long periods of time or heavy lifting): _____

_____

My hobbies (including sports): _____

_____

My exercise regimen: _____

_____

Current tobacco, alcohol or illicit drug use: ___

_____

## A Slave to Bed Rest

The pain was all too familiar. It started in my lower right back, then took on a life of its own. Before I knew it, sitting at work was tortuous. Driving my car was excruciating.

I actually felt lucky. Lucky? Yes—my back had survived two pregnancies (natural deliveries, mind you) and twenty years since my last battle of the bulging disc. The memories are bittersweet.

The first time around, I was 20-something and married only a few years. This was before the advent of the Internet, but I read everything I could on back pain. By the time I dragged myself to the doctor, I knew what my diagnosis would be. I also knew that what my mother had drilled into my head all those years was true: Good posture is important. (Okay, Mom, you can say "I told you so.")

In those days, back injuries were treated differently. The first doctor I visited recommended the "s" word (surgery), and I quickly—as quickly as someone whose back is in spasm can manage—found another doctor. He prescribed ten weeks of bed rest (yes, ten weeks!), plus physical therapy (PT). No pain medication. Ouch.

This is where the memories start kicking in. You see, my husband was the lucky guy who chauffeured me from the suburbs to the city three days a week for PT. Plus put in a full day's work. On Mondays, Wednesdays and Fridays, his schedule went like this: Drive Darcy to PT. Wait for Darcy at PT. Watch the physical therapist ask Darcy what number, on a scale of 1 to 10 (10 being worst), her pain was on that given day. Listen as Darcy replied, through gritted teeth, "Ten." Watch Darcy get put on a torture rack (translation: traction machine). I think he secretly may have gotten a little perverse pleasure out of that one.

His day continued: Drive Darcy home from PT. Drive back into the city for work. Drive home from work. That added up to two hours of driving daily. It's a miracle his back didn't give out!

Or his patience, for that matter. You see, I was only allowed out of bed for "necessities." I was obsessed by the thought that being confined to bed would cause me to balloon like a sumo wrestler. So I put myself on a strict diet. Of course, my husband was the caterer. And how he catered to me! Half a grapefruit for breakfast. Salad for lunch. A balanced dinner. No snacks. No sweets. No fun.

As my therapy progressed, I was allowed to go

swimming. After all, swimming is weightless and puts no stress on the back. No one mentioned the stress it can put on one's spouse who has to accompany you to the swim club.

After weeks of grapefruit and salad, I must admit I didn't look too bad in my swimsuit. That is, if you could get past the fact that I shuffled along like my poor old Aunt Ruthie.

Once I was in the pool, it was like heaven. My pain and worries literally floated away. So did my wedding band.

You see, I really had lost weight during this ordeal. So much so, that apparently my rings were now loose on my fingers. If only I'd noticed this before I took the plunge into the deep end of the pool. There I was, clinging to the side of the pool, looking down at a glimmer of gold that seemed perilously close to the drain.

Throughout my entire rehabilitation, I never once cried or felt sorry for myself. I just dealt with it. Period. Well, I must have had enough bottled-up emotions to fill an entire season of modern-day "Dr. Phil" shows, because the floodgates burst. I sobbed so hard and so long that I think the chlorinated water became saltwater.

My fully dressed husband stood helplessly on the pool deck, shaking his head in disbelief.

As luck would have it, a scuba diving class was

being held in the shallow end of the Olympic-sized pool. We explained the situation—undoubtedly providing much more medical history than necessary—and, in a flash of bubbles, fins and masks, my precious wedding band was retrieved.

Wondering how I dealt with my most recent bout with my stubborn disc? Physical therapy, low-heeled shoes and perfect posture. That, and the realization that my loving husband might just go on strike if I so much as mentioned the words "bed rest."

To this day, my husband reminds me of how he was my "slave" for those ten weeks. He even painted my toenails for me. If that's not true love, I don't know what is. It's no wonder I almost "lost it" when I almost lost my wedding band in the pool that day.

♥ *Darcy Silvers*

# You've Got a
# Lot of Nerve: Sciatica

If you're like many people, when you experience a pain that goes down one leg, your immediate thought is, "I've got sciatica!" But let's get a couple of misconceptions out of the way: Not every pain that radiates down the leg is sciatica—and sciatica is a symptom of other snafus, not a diagnosis in itself.

Sciatica is pain caused by inflammation or compression of the sciatic nerve, which, as we mentioned earlier, runs from the lower back down the back of each leg. You may experience a pain in the rear (though you may *think* that this is caused by your boss or kids); pain or a burning or tingling sensation that runs down one leg; or a weakness or numbness of the leg or foot—or even all of the above at the same time!

While the most common cause of sciatica is a lumbar herniated disc (also called a *slipped disc* or *ruptured disc*), other causes of this symptom include degenerative disc disease, bone spurs (a bony growth formed on natural bone), lumbar spinal stenosis (where part of the spinal canal narrows, putting pressure on the sciatic nerve) or piriformis syndrome (where the muscle that runs directly above the sciatic nerve puts pressure on the sciatic nerve).

## Getting Diagnosed

Your health-care provider needs to figure out if you indeed have sciatica—that is, whether the sciatic nerve is inflamed or something is putting pressure on it—and if so, pinpoint which part of the nerve is affected. To do this, he'll first take your medical history and perform a physical exam. He may also test your muscle strength, sensation and reflexes, or ask you to perform movements such as walking on your heels or toes. Another test that identifies sciatic pain involves sitting in a chair, extending one leg, raising it, then repeating the process with the other leg.

If your pain is very severe or doesn't improve within six weeks, your health-care provider may recommend imaging tests such as X-rays or an MRI to find out whether the sciatic nerve is being compressed by a disc, bone spurs, infection, fractures or tumors and to rule out other possible causes of the pain. (See page 69 for more on X-rays, MRIs and other diagnostic tools.)

## Deep-Sixing Sciatica

The good news about sciatica—strange though that phrase may sound—is that roughly 95 percent of people with sciatica get better without the need for surgery. In one study, two groups of patients were treated for sciatica: one surgically, the other medically. At the beginning of the study, the surgical group fared better, but after six months, both groups fared equally well, with no difference in outcome!

With that in mind, here are techniques for putting the kibosh on sciatica if you already suffer from it:

- Manual treatments like physical therapy and chiropractic can relieve the pressure on the nerve if you suffer from acute back injury or sciatica.

- A nonsteroidal anti-inflammatory drug (NSAID) may help alleviate the inflammation and pain of sciatica. See chapter 10 for more on NSAIDs and other medications.

- For acute pain, try applying a cold pack to the painful areas for 20 to 30 minutes, repeating every two hours or as needed for up to 48 hours. After 48 hours of using a cold pack, apply a heating pad to the painful area for 20 to 30 minutes; repeat every two hours as needed. (If you have chronic pain, stick with heat and avoid the cold compress.) Inspect your skin frequently with both hot and cold packs to make sure the extreme temperatures aren't damaging your skin.

• Ask your doctor for stretching exercises that can help relieve the pain. Your physical therapist can also give you stretches to try, and you can also try the stretches on page 19.

• If your health-care provider is skilled in pain management, she may prescribe epidural steroid injections to reduce inflammation and relieve pressure on the sciatic nerve.

• Surgery is a serious step, and thankfully most sufferers of sciatica will get better without it. But if you and your doctor decide that this course of action will be best for you, you may undergo a *microdiscectomy* or *lumbar laminectomy* and *discectomy,* where the surgeon removes the portion of the disc that's irritating the nerve root. Surgery is meant to prevent permanent nerve damage and may not cure your back pain, so be sure to talk to your doctor and get a second (or even a third) opinion. Check out page 89 for more information on surgery.

## Think about . . .
### my symptoms

Taking stock of my symptoms will help my health-care provider diagnose my back pain. I have:

\_\_ Lower back pain.

\_\_ Pain that runs down the back of one or both of my legs.

\_\_ Pain that runs from the midbuttock down the back of one leg to the knee. (If the pain stops at the knee, it may not be sciatica.)

\_\_ Pain that runs down the outside of the calf and the top of the foot, ending between the last two toes or in the big toe. (Different nerve roots will lead to pain in different parts of the feet.)

\_\_ Pain that runs down the inside of the calf and behind the ankle to the sole of the foot.

\_\_ A tingling or burning sensation that runs down one leg.

\_\_ A feeling of weakness or numbness in the leg or foot.

## From Back Pain to Backbends

My back pain changed my life.

It started in my right arm and spread to my wrist and middle finger. However, the source of the throbbing was a pinched nerve in my spine. I couldn't lift everyday items or hold my toddler. I couldn't open jars or pull weeds. Sitting was unbearable. Lying down was worse.

This was seven months ago. Just before the pain surfaced, I was an anxious, stressed-out mom who screamed at her children: a boy, five, and a girl, two. My husband was away in Iraq for the second time in a year.

I didn't want to be mean and grumpy. I had hoped to be more relaxed and achieve more during this deployment. During my husband's first time in Iraq, I lost my sanity and was sure he would not return, especially after he was wounded. I was scatter-brained, losing my keys, leaving the lights on in the car. I even closed the car trunk on my head, which resulted in four stitches.

This time, I wouldn't lose my cool. I would be calm, efficient. I had planned projects for the house and for my work.

Looking back now, I realize I was aiming for an ideal that wasn't necessary. There was no reason to always be happy or try to control things beyond my reach. These unrealistic goals would cause me mental anguish and eventually physical pain.

It had been about eight weeks since my husband had left for Iraq when I awoke one morning and couldn't turn my neck. There were shooting pains down my forearm and tingling in my fingers.

I was irritated by the pain, annoyed that one more thing was getting in the way of my perfectly laid plans for a successful deployment. The pain was excruciating and the only way to make it go away—and this sounds strange—was to raise my hand in the air, like I was waiting to be called on to answer a question in school. Despite this, I was sure the pain would go away later that day, if not the next. It didn't.

A friend drove me to my doctor's office. He recommended pain pills and muscle relaxants. I was told to return in a week. I didn't think I would need anything after that, but the pain got worse.

The second time I saw the doctor he ordered an MRI and started talking about neurologists and surgery. He gave me a splint for my arm, thinking I had carpel tunnel syndrome. He told me to stop writing because it aggravated my symptoms.

That's when I knew it was bad. Writing was my life. I didn't mind the practical setbacks, like not being able to pull weeds, but I could not imagine my life without expressing myself on paper.

The MRI confirmed a large bulge on my upper spine. I had a bulging disc, more commonly known as a pinched nerve. I began to research back ailments such as mine. I wanted to get well—soon.

I saw a physical therapist three times a week and within six weeks was off the drugs and was cleared to start yoga. By this time I began to understand that back pain doesn't affect only the frail and elderly or construction workers, or those with a bad back with poor exercise habits. My yoga teacher taught me that bad backs happen especially to those who have stress and anxiety in their lives.

I gradually realized the prescription for my healthy back: let go of the stress to be the perfect do-it-all mom while my husband was away; let go of grandiose writing plans, for the time being anyway; stop worrying about a husband in Fallujah who might not return; and do yoga at least twice a week. I followed this regimen for five months.

A few weeks ago I did my first backbend ever in my life.

The ground shifted beneath my head as I arched

up from the ground. I saw the sky behind me get a little closer. I kept pushing and I felt the swoosh of air under my head. I was up. I was doing a back-bend. I held it there—breathless.

Although I had been symptom-free for several months, achieving that backbend was a turning point for me. My body was strong, flexible and pliable. But more importantly, I had learned not to aim for unrealistic, broad goals, but rather to focus on one thing at a time, such as achieving the arch and the lift of the backbend.

These days I laugh with my children, play soccer with them and pull them in the wagon. I can sit at my desk and write (and accomplish more in less time). My anxiety has disappeared. Oh, and my yard is weed-free.

♥ *Ingrid Bairstow*

# No Bones About It: Osteoporosis

We don't think about our bones very much. We'd be pretty floppy without them, but we don't even consider our bones until something happens to them—like they become weak and brittle.

Weak, brittle bones are caused by a condition called osteoporosis, which occurs when the body's process for removing old bone and replacing it with new bone gets out of whack. When bone material is *resorbed* (that is, broken down) too quickly or replaced too slowly, your bones become weak and at risk for fractures.

Osteoporosis can make your back hurt by causing fractures of the vertebrae, and osteoporosis causes roughly 700,000 vertebral fractures annually. That's a lot of fractures! While one-third of these fractures cause pain, the majority of them produce no symptoms at all.

In the U.S., ten million people—eight million women and two million men—have osteoporosis, and 34 million more are at risk of osteoporosis due to low bone mass. (These numbers will likely rise dramatically in the years ahead as members of the baby boom generation ease into senior-citizen status.) Fifty percent of women over age 50 and 25 percent of men over age 50 will have an osteoporosis-related fracture in their lifetime.

The causes of osteoporosis are numerous, and many of the risk factors can't be changed or eliminated. When women enter menopause, for example, they start producing fewer estrogen hormones, which prevent osteoporosis. (This is why doctors sometimes prescribe estrogen or progesterone replacement therapy to women to reduce the risk of osteoporosis.)

Other unpreventable risk factors are being Caucasian or Asian or having a family history of the condition. For men, low testosterone levels are a common cause of osteoporosis.

But not every cause of osteoporosis is set in genetic stone. Here are several preventable risk factors that can cause bone thinning:

- Low calcium and vitamin D intake.
- A couch potato lifestyle.
- Smoking.
- Excessive alcohol intake.
- Long-term use of glucocorticoids, certain cancer treatments and/or certain anticonvulsants.
- Anorexia.

Many people don't know they have osteoporosis until a bone fracture brings it to light, but bone mineral density (BMD) tests can spot osteoporosis before a fracture brings you the bad news. Your doctor may order a BMD test if you have multiple risk factors for osteoporosis. (See page 72 for the scoop on this test.)

## The Calcium Connection

Many of us know that calcium plays an important role in maintaining healthy bone mass. So why do national surveys show that many of us consume less than half the recommended amount? Check out the sidebar for information on how much calcium you need daily, and try these tips for getting more calcium in your diet.

- **Down the dairy.** Milk and other dairy products provide the best sources for calcium, and three daily servings of dairy provides all the calcium you need. And good news for dieters: skim milk actually contains more calcium than whole milk.

- **Look past milk.** Sure, dairy products have calcium, but so do other foods, such as broccoli, almonds, tofu, spinach, and sardines and salmon with bones. To find out the calcium content of your favorite foods, visit the U.S. Department of Agriculture's Nutrient Data Laboratory Web site at *www.nal.usda.gov/fnic/foodcomp*.

- **If you're lactose intolerant,** try a specialized

product such as Lactaid brand milk. Many people with lactose intolerance can also handle hard cheese and yogurt without stomach upset.

- **Look for calcium-fortified foods like orange juice and cereal.**

- **Put powdered milk in the mix.** A tablespoon of nonfat powdered dry milk boasts 52 milligrams of calcium, and you can add it to puddings, homemade baked goods, cooked cereal, soups, gravy and other foods.

- **If you don't get enough calcium from your food,** take calcium supplements, whether they're calcium carbonate (such as Tums) or calcium citrate. It's better to split up your supplementation so you take half in the morning and half at night. (If you have kidney stones, consult your doctor before taking calcium supplements.) The recommended amounts for calcium refer to elemental calcium, so just make sure you get enough elemental calcium from these supplements.

- **Gimme a D.** Since vitamin D helps the body absorb calcium, experts recommend consuming between 400 and 800 IU (international units) daily. Vitamin D is manufactured in the skin in response to exposure to sunlight, but the skin's ability to make vitamin D decreases with age. Major food sources of this vitamin are egg yolks, vitamin D-fortified dairy products, liver and saltwater fish. Most multi-vitamins contain vitamin D as well.

## Move It or Lose It

Just like muscle, bone becomes stronger when you exercise it. Both weight-bearing and resistance exercises can help build and maintain bone mass.

Resistance exercises are those that build muscle strength, such as weight lifting. Weight-bearing exercises are those where you're supporting your own body weight: think walking, jogging, stair climbing or even standing (if you stand four hours or so each day). The exercise needs to have some degree of impact; cycling and swimming, for example, are not weight-bearing exercises.

Check with your doctor before beginning any exercise program. With his okay, you can find exercises you enjoy.

## Never Too Late

If you already have osteoporosis, your health-care provider may prescribe a medication that can help build bone mass, such as alendronate (Fosamax), residronate (Actonel) or ibandronate

(Boniva), which are all in the same family of drugs called bisphosphonates. Other medications include raloxifene (Evista), which is only for women, and teriparatide (Forteo), which is intended for high-risk patients. The list of approved medications is long, and your doctor will take your risk factors into account when prescribing one.

## Your Daily Dose

This is how many milligrams of calcium you should be consuming every day, according to the National Academy of Sciences.

| | |
|---|---|
| Birth to 6 months | 210 |
| 6 months to 1 year | 270 |
| 1–3 | 500 |
| 4–8 | 800 |
| 9–13 | 1300 |
| 14–18 | 1300 |
| 19–30 | 1000 |
| 31–50 | 1000 |
| 51–70 | 1200 |
| 70 or older | 1200 |

## Think about . . .
## preventing osteoporosis

These are the things I can do to start preventing osteoporosis today:

\_\_ Eat more dairy products such as lowfat milk, yogurt, nonfat dried milk powder and cheese.

\_\_ Choose calcium-fortified cereal, orange juice and bread.

\_\_ Eat more nondairy foods that naturally contain calcium such as spinach, almonds and broccoli.

\_\_ Eat more foods that contain vitamin D such as egg yolks, vitamin D-fortified dairy products, liver and saltwater fish.

\_\_ Take calcium supplements (if I don't get enough calcium from my diet).

\_\_ Start doing resistance exercises like weight lifting. (I'll consult with my doctor first.)

\_\_ Start doing weight-bearing exercises like walking, jogging, stair climbing or dancing. (I'll consult with my doctor first.)

\_\_ Quit smoking.

\_\_ Decrease my alcohol consumption.

\_\_ Talk to my doctor about minimizing the intake of meds that can cause bone loss.

## Back to Normal

The sign on the door reads, "Please enter quietly." Although no sound issues from my lips, every muscle fiber in my back screams, sending painful rays throughout my entire body. I turn the doorknob and, after brief hesitation, softly cross the threshold, hoping this time I'll finally find relief.

From the start, I sense that this massage therapy could be different. For almost 30 minutes, Roseanne issues questions about past injuries, physical activity level, eating and work habits, ergonomics and family history. More thorough than any medical doctor I'd seen, she covers an entire lifetime of possible triggers for the back pain that haunts me.

So here I lie, still somewhat apprehensive, but warm and comfortable under the weight of a heated blanket. As barely audible notes from a CD player fill the sandalwood-scented air, I close my eyes and attempt to relax. My previous unsuccessful experiences—prescription medication, acupuncture, body balancing, chiropractic and

physical therapy—swim through my brain as I
wonder what this latest endeavor will bring.

Roseanne begins by gliding hot, smooth stones
over my aching muscles. Each time her capable
hands detect areas of misalignment, she cautiously
works the muscles until they relent. Now and then
during the session, I hear and feel a "pop," which
produces a welcome release along with Roseanne's
explanation of what just occurred. Although I am
somewhat familiar with basic human anatomy, my
medical education is enhanced as I lie on that massage table.

Suddenly, Roseanne's voice breaks the quiet in
the room. "Now I want you to push your knee
against the palm of my hand when I give the signal."

What's this? Roseanne is asking me to participate actively in the therapy? All my previous therapeutic experiences never required my personal
involvement. In fact, I often felt removed from the
process. Puzzled, but desperate to ease the pain, I
obey her request. Slowly, and surprisingly, the
tightness in my back releases as I exert pressure
against her palm. Keep breathing, she reminds me.
I'm so absorbed in my efforts to comply, I don't
realize I am holding my breath.

At various times throughout the remainder of
the hour-long session, I respond to instructions to
bend, flex, lift, pull and straighten. By the time my

massage is complete, I feel mentally and physically energized as if I've just finished a vigorous workout.

With follow-up appointment card in hand, I'm preparing to leave the office when Roseanne's voice stops my progress. "I want you to perform these exercises at home every night before you go to bed." Now she's giving me homework? Too surprised to speak, I take the printed handout, smile, and exit.

That evening I scan the sheet and follow the directions for some inner and outer thigh exercises intended to strengthen muscles that connect and support my lumbar spine. Roseanne's in-office treatment helped work out a few kinks. Maybe the at-home supplemental therapy will help as well, I think.

Two weeks later, after faithfully completing my homework, I return to Roseanne's office feeling only slightly better. She asks for an update on my condition and then begins the session. At this, and the next several meetings, she "listens" to my body as she works, continually informing me of her strategy and imparting valuable information about the interconnectedness of muscles and how she hopes to help me.

Our conversations reverberate even when I am not on the massage table. At my desk, grocery shopping, driving the car or sitting in a movie theater, I recall her words regarding posture, alignment and breathing. After a couple of weeks, I find that unconsciously I heed her advice and that, surprisingly, back pain no longer consumes me every minute of the day. While still plagued with some morning stiffness and nighttime aches, my days have become relatively pain free.

After three months of therapy, I find that I can roll out of bed without fearing the sharp pain that greeted my mornings for so long. Bending down to retrieve a dropped object no longer elicits that familiar twinge.

More valuable than Roseanne's knowledge, skill, resolve and commitment is my own engagement in the therapeutic process. Thanks to her encouragement, I feel more in control and grow increasingly aware of the way I carry myself and move my body. This collaboration of efforts is something different and new to me. Roseanne not only facilitated physical healing through her proficiency and persistence, but also provided emotional support and genuine interest in my well-being.

I continue to schedule monthly massages with Roseanne as preventive maintenance. Now when I cross that threshold though, I know exactly what I'll find on the other side.

♥ *Phyllis Hanlon*

# The Great Imitators

When is back pain not back pain?

When it's kidney stones, back labor, endometriosis, gallstones . . .

It sounds like a joke, but the punch line isn't so funny: what feels like a pain in your back can actually be a symptom of a condition in another part of the body. (Thankfully, in the vast majority of cases back pain isn't a symptom of a serious condition.) Here are some possible causes of back pain that's not really back pain:

- **Urinary tract infections**

    Urinary tract infections (UTIs), which are caused by bacteria in the urinary tract, can cause pain in the lower back (which really comes from the kidneys), among other symptoms.

- **Gallstones**

    The gallbladder stores a liquid called bile, which is used to help the body digest fats. Gallstones form when bile hardens into pieces of stonelike material, and these faux stones can cause a pain between the shoulder blades as a symptom.

## • Endometriosis

Endometriosis is a chronic condition where tissue from the uterus is found elsewhere in the body—for example, on the ovaries, the fallopian tubes or the lining of the pelvic cavity. This condition, which affects 5.5 million girls and women in the U.S. and Canada, can cause lower back pain as one of its symptoms.

## • Back labor

Back labor is a lower back pain (or hip pain) that's caused when the about-to-be-born fetus moves face up through the birth canal instead of face down.

## • Vitamin C overdose

Overdose of vitamin C is rare, but one of its symptoms is back pain.

## • Kidney stones

What do you get when a hard material forms out of substances in the urine? A kidney stone. The stone may stay in the kidney or travel down the urinary tract. If the stone is large, it can get stuck in a ureter, the bladder or the urethra and cause back pain as one of its symptoms.

### • Drug side effects

Back pain is a side effect of certain allergy medicines, statin drugs (which are used to lower cholesterol) and other medications.

Your health-care provider will perform a thorough physical to get to the root of your back pain—whether it's a back injury, one of these conditions or something else. To help her diagnose you, be sure to note any other symptoms you have, include a list of every drug you take (whether prescription or over the counter) and detail your family health history.

## Red Flags

Fewer than 5 percent of patients with back pain have a serious condition. However, in rare cases, back pain can be a symptom of a serious problem such as heart attack, cancer, pneumonia, blood clot in the lung or peptic ulcer disease.

To rule out more serious conditions, you should see a doctor immediately if you experience fever, drastic weight loss, numbness down one or both legs, weakness of the legs, pain at rest or pain that keeps you from sleeping, or loss of bladder or bowel control.

# Dodging the Indoor Hammer

February 1, 2002. Virginia Military Institute hosted its annual winter indoor track and field meet. Southern Virginia University, a small college of 500 students, fielded its very first track and field team. There I stood in the track infield watching two of my boys running the 200-meter dash. The gun went off and suddenly I felt an explosion of pain in my neck and back. The force of the blow sent me careening to the floor and momentarily I knew the eerie sensation of passing fluidly from consciousness to unconsciousness.

What had happened? Surely, the starter had not shot real bullets out of the gun. The mystery revealed itself as I caught movement from the corner of my eye. A competitor in the 35-pound weight throw competition stammered a semblance of an apology as members of the athletic training staff hovered around me. Moments earlier I had been standing sandwiched between two of my waiflike girl athletes, the next moment I tasted the rubbery surface of the VMI track. Evidently, an indoor hammer had been tossed twenty feet outside of the sector. The velocity of the hammer combined with its weight and trajectory was enough to fell a small buffalo, let alone a lanky cross-country coach.

After this incident, Coach Wright was a pitiful sight on campus and even more pitiful at practice. No longer able to demonstrate how to pole vault, hurdle, high jump or throw the shot, I suddenly had to rely on the voice of experience rather than the body. The spring semester was a testimony to personal frustration.

As a teacher of sports psychology, I have come to the conclusion that people deal with injuries much like they handle the death of a loved one. The first stage of the grieving process is denial. Indeed, I laughed off to my athletes the idea that I was hurt or in any way less capable than I wanted to be. Consequently, I still attempted to run with my team, coach by example, play in intramurals and on the whole make no real attempt at careful rehabilitation. I did not want to admit to being less than whole, so I denied my injury its true status.

The second stage of the grief process is anger. Boy, did I get cross at myself, my injury and at times everyone else around me. At times, I even blamed the dog for my injury. One time, one of my athletes threw a shot and it almost hit a teammate.

The throw was uncontrolled but not at all a deliberate attempt to brain her friend. The poor athlete in question got a mouthful from me, which later made us both feel bad, and then I followed it up by picking up a girl's shot and demonstrating correct technique. This "correct technique" caused the shot to fly across the gym and straight through the exterior paneled wall. Added to the damage was the daggerlike pain that coursed through my spinal cord. Practice ended early and I limped off to my office to lie down on the floor until the spasms ceased.

The third stage of the grieving process is bargaining. I became a great negotiator. My true love is running and the back injury broke my running heart. So as painful as it was, I started to be good for three days so I could enjoy the endorphin-release of a trail run on the fourth day. I did not enjoy taking time out for treatment and rehabilitation, but I did so as a trade-off for being able to participate in some form of physical activity.

The fourth stage of the grieving process is depression. Boy, did I live this stage to the fullest. Many of my dearest friends swore that they saw a little rain cloud following me everywhere I went. I started to lose weight, my appetite disappeared, I continued to toss and turn at night, I felt hopeless, and no amount of chocolate chip cookies could cheer me up. We won the National Small School's track and field championship later that year. The celebratory dinner might as well have been a wake for all the happiness it brought me. Yes, my athletes had succeeded, but poor little Coach could not throw a javelin in a straight line, could not serve a tennis ball and had no chance of swimming a lick of freestyle.

The fifth stage of the grieving process is acceptance. The true day of acceptance arrived in early May. The day of the Iron-man came and went. The previous year of training lay beside the road unused and wasted. I searched online for the results and pined and cried a few silent tears. A friend had given me Dan Millman's book, *How to Succeed in Sport & Life.* I sat in my office and opened it. It fell open at a random page on which was written a quote from Henry David Thoreau:

*"If one advances confidently in the direction of his dreams, and endeavors to live the life which he has imagined, he will meet with a success unexpected in common hours."*

I realized in that moment that the grieving process needed to be over. The agonizing, sometimes debilitating back pain was forcing me to live a life incongruent with my dreams and far removed from what I imagined it would be. It was time to seek out success in the common hours.

Immediately, I started to treat my back pain as a mental and emotional limitation. I grew more positive about the exercises of my rehabilitation. Knowing that lower back pain is also symptomatic of five primary physical problems (a weak lower back, stiff lower back, tight hamstrings, tight quadriceps and weak abdominal muscles), I began to take ownership for my recovery. I set goals again. Five months out from the trauma, I completed the Nashville Country Music Marathon. Not the fastest race I had ever run, definitely not the most comfortable, but perhaps one of the most rewarding.

With this new zest for life and a goal-driven energy, my body almost miraculously began to heal itself. In the weight room, I grew stronger. Suddenly, I was able to pick up my two-year-old daughter again and swing her around in the air. In the next two years, I continued to set new goals. I went to Africa and climbed Kilimanjaro, I backpacked a major portion of the Appalachian Trail. I ran several more marathons and competed in a number of short triathlons. I continued coaching and training with my athletes. I even went to two coaching clinics to learn how better to coach the indoor hammer.

The doctors informed me that the likelihood is that I shall always have pain in my back. The scar tissue will never completely disappear and the unevenness of my shoulder blades is a constant reminder of an unkind projectile. There is also the suggestion that a little bit of arthritis has crept into the once-traumatized area. Like a barometer, my back lets me know the weather forecast. In the cold, I remain wooden and stiff. Before subjecting my racquetball students to an unruly defeat, I find I must warm my back up with "yogaesque" stretching. I refuse to let the pain beat me and I refuse to just lie down and let life pass me by. For indeed as Jack London, the famous author, cries, "The purpose of man is to live, not exist."

♥ *Dr. Paul Wright*

# We Can See Right Through You: Diagnostic Tools

Here's a story about the power of names. In 1895, W. C. Roentgen invented roentgenograms. If the name had stuck, we would have grown up buying Roentgen-specs from comic book ads and Superman would have had Roentgen vision. But thankfully, what were once called roentgenograms are now called by a much catchier (and easier to pronounce) name: X-rays.

If your back hurts, your health-care provider may order tests such as X-rays as well as MRIs, PET scans, bone scans, bone mineral density tests or CAT scans, depending on what he suspects is wrong.

"Yikes!" you say. "You mean I have to wear one of those lead bibs and crawl inside a machine?" Never fear—here, we'll tell you what these scans are, when your doctor is likely to use them and what you can expect.

- **X-rays**

    The process sounds like an invention from a science fiction novel: X-rays are radiated through a particular body part (such as your back). Tissues of different densities absorb different amounts of the radiation—bones, for example, absorb the most radiation, so they appear whiter in the final image. X-rays can detect structural problems in your back such as fractures, slipped vertebrae, narrow disc spaces, calcium deposits, spurs and even kidney stones and gallstones!

The radiologist (the professional who takes X-rays) may cover nonaffected parts of your body with a lead apron to protect them from radiation. Then she'll position you on a table. You'll be asked to remain still and hold your breath for a few seconds while the radiologist takes the X-ray.

• **MRIs**

An MRI (magnetic resonance imaging) uses huge magnets that rotate around the body to show the relationship between the various parts of your back—in 256 shades of gray! The MRI scan displays your anatomy by showing the contrast between tissues that contain a lot of water (such as discs or cerebrospinal fluid) and those that contain little water (like nerve roots or bone). MRIs are especially useful for determining whether your back pain is coming from a nerve that's being compressed by a disc. MRIs can also help rule out infections or tumors.

You know that magnets attract metal, so it probably comes as no surprise that people with metallic objects like a pacemaker in their bodies can't get an MRI. Some types of metal aren't affected by the MRI, so if you're positive that you know what's inside, ask the MRI technician if you can be scanned safely.

When you get an MRI, you'll lie on a motorized table that carries you slowly into the machine. You'll need to lie still until the MRI is complete, which can take up to an hour. The test is painless and you're lying comfortably on the table. If being enclosed in tight spaces gives you the jitters, you can either search for a facility that uses "open" scanners, which some find more tolerable, or talk with your doctor about being sedated.

• **Bone Scans**

A bone scan can show tumors, infections, fractures and other back woes in bony tissue. To do the scan, the technician injects a radiotracer into a vein, and this tracer is taken up into actively inflamed bones. The radiotracer gives off gamma radiation as it decays, and a camera can detect this gamma radiation during the scan.

The most difficult thing about a bone scan is that the radiotracer takes two to three hours to reach the inflamed bone. (Hope you brought a book with you!) Once the tracer is in place, the technician will take an hour or so to perform the scan. As for the radiation, it decays quickly and passes completely from your body after two to three days. The amount of radiation you receive is usually less than what you get from a chest X-ray.

• **CAT Scan**

Using X-ray beams that rotate around the patient, a CAT (computed axial tomography) scan—also known as a CT (computed tomography) scan—gives your doctor a three-dimensional view of a part of your anatomy in cross-sectional slices. It can show both soft tissues and bone, and helps your doctor diagnose herniated discs, fractures and other spinal problems.

As with an MRI scan, you'll lie on a motorized table. The table slowly carries you into the scanner, then the scanner rotates around your body, emitting low-intensity X-ray beams. You'll need to lie still for the few minutes that the test takes, and you face no chance of turning into the Hulk or Spiderman.

• **Bone Mineral Density Test**

A bone mineral density (BMD) test measures the amount of the mineral calcium in certain bones: the more calcium, the denser the bone. The BMD shows whether you have (or are at risk for) osteoporosis, and your doctor may order the test if you have risk factors such as being postmenopausal or being on long-term corticosteroid therapy. The two types of BMD tests are the quantitative CT scan that uses a CT scanner (like the one we just described) and the DXA test, a type of X-ray that's the gold standard of bone tests at this time and ideal for at-risk patients.

The results of your test are reported in T-scores and Z-scores. For postmenopausal women, the T-score compares your bone density to a premenopausal woman's average peak bone density; for men, the T-score compares your bone density to a younger man's peak bone density. A score above -1 indicates normal bone density; -1 to -2.5 means you have low bone density and are at risk of osteoporosis; and below -2.5 shows that you already have osteoporosis. (The score reading may vary if you're a woman of color or a man since your bone density tends to be higher than that of postmenopausal white women.) If you've already sustained a *fragility fracture* (a compression fracture), then by definition you have osteoporosis and the DXA score isn't needed for a diagnosis. However, you might want to have the DXA done to monitor response to treatment.

The Z-score compares your test results to what's normally expected for someone of your weight, sex, age and ethnicity. Based on your risk factors and the density results, your doctor will decide whether or not you need to be treated for osteoporosis.

• **PET Scan**

Unlike a bone scan, a positron emission tomography (PET) scan looks primarily at soft tissues. A PET scan shows both organ structure and function and can be used to detect disease, tumors and other medical problems.

To start, the technician injects a small amount of radiotracer into a vein. After sixty minutes or so, the radiotracer will accumulate in a certain part of the body, depending on where you were injected. You then lie on a motorized table that slowly brings you through the scanner. The PET scan detects the energy given off by the radiotracer, and a computer converts the energy into three-dimensional pictures. The process takes about 45 minutes, and you need to lie still while the test takes place.

## Studying for the Test

Here are questions you may want to ask your doctor before undergoing a test:

- What sort of preparation will I need for this test? (You may need to remove metal objects such as jewelry or refrain from eating for a certain amount of time before the test.)
- Can I undergo this test if I'm pregnant?
- Can I undergo this test if I have a metallic implant?
- Will I be injected with a contrast agent (which enhances the images)? If I have kidney disease, how will this contrast agent affect my kidneys? (Also, alert the technician if you have a history of contrast dye allergy.)
- How long should the test take?
- What kinds of conditions does this test detect?

## Studying for the Test (cont'd)

- Will my insurance plan pay for this test? (All of these tests are expensive, and while they won't be ordered willy-nilly, you should know ahead of time who's footing the bill.)
- Is there anything else I should know?

## *Not Born to Run*

Running wasn't something I ever thought I'd do. In graduate school, however, my boyfriend was a runner, and my best friend ran. I also had a fantastically athletic German-short-haired pointer named Moxie, who required serious exercise.

I started with very short distances. Moxie could have happily gone 30 times further, and my pace kept me only a nose ahead of pedestrians, but moving my body outside with a smiling Moxie was a wonderful break from studying and fretting.

Then I met Sophie, a professional runner also cuckoo in-love with her dog, Ginger. To my surprise, Sophie offered to coach me. She devised schedules and met me for weekly workouts. She even ran with me! Nobody else wanted to run with slowpoke. Sophie took me seriously, and out of gratitude I did too. I grew stronger and faster. Moxie thrived, and I fretted less.

While running I first experienced joy. I don't mean happiness, but something more profound. My keenest memory comes from a summer spent running outside a little Oregon town. Moxie and I regularly ran to a nearby lake, swam and ran back. On the way, we passed through evergreens, old orchards and fields of golden grass. Here I felt a chest-expanding feeling, almost painful, which I could only release with a laugh. The world seemed abundant and benign, and I had place in it. And this was enough.

The trouble began when I took a desk job. And since I was writing my dissertation, I also sat before a computer at home. Soon I was in pain. It originated where my spine meets my hips, and shot below one buttock and down my leg. The pain was insistent and intensified over the week. By the end of each day all I could do was lie down, and by week's end, I was tearful and desperate.

My doctor was blunt.

"If you want to ruin your back, keep running."

I had always appreciated Dr. Veneta's frankness, but she had never been so stern.

"I know from experience that runners ignore me," she continued. "But your back isn't made for running."

I was hoping for a therapy referral, not a terminal diagnosis. But I wasn't surprised. A number of years ago, another doctor had been almost rude: "You're not put together very well."

Both doctors were referring to my scoliosis, a lateral curvature of the spine that tends to throw the whole body off. People with scoliosis shouldn't run since pounding the pavement is hard on a spine whose misaligned vertebrae do not stack neatly when compressed.

I learned of my scoliosis at thirteen. After touching my toes several times during a screening, I heard the teacher stage whisper, "Should we tell her?" The curve wasn't pronounced enough to warrant a brace. The doctor concluded that only time would tell if trouble would develop.

In my midthirties, time told.

As Dr. Veneta predicted, I kept running, but I also went to physical therapy. The PT diagnosed me with a bulging disc. His treatment was to push the vertebrae apart to relieve pressure and persuade the disc to return home. But there was a lot of tissue between his hands and my vertebrae, and sometimes I bruised. It soon became clear: the treatment was failing. I decided to give up running.

While the pain became more manageable, my weight and mood became less so. Plus, my Guilt-O-Meter was always in the red with Moxie. At night I dreamed of running, of breath and muscle and speed. I felt the wind against my face, and then, still dreaming, I remembered that I wasn't supposed to run anymore. Sadness replaced exhilaration as I broke stride.

For several years I sought a replacement for running and managed my pain as best I could. Then I heard of a physical therapist who healed what others couldn't. When I called, Melinda asked some questions and assessed my condition. "That's a pretty easy fix."

Sure.

To reach Melinda's, I drove for miles, turned up a gravel road and parked at the woods' edge. A short path led to an office in the trees. She examined me and confirmed her hunch: A torsion in my hips. The spine passes through them, and having one hip tilted forward causes pain from sitting, walking and running. While Melinda gently manipulated my body, I gazed into the woods and listened to the birds' lovely racket. She showed me some simple exercises and sent me on my way.

The whole experience had a fairy-tale quality. Melinda the Good Witch, I would say, Melinda the Good. I later learned that others, even other PTs, called her similar things. The healing, however, was quite real; the pain was gone. After three visits, Melinda said I could run again.

Now when I run my steady, never speedy pace, Moxie darts through the high grass, sometimes flushing pheasant. The other day she startled a turkey into the air just above my head. Melinda tells me that because of my scoliosis I must avoid heavy mileage. That's fine. Three glorious miles every other day is enough.

♥ *Hilary Hart*

# Hands-On Treatment

Maybe the treatment for your back woes sounds like "snap, crackle, pop." Or perhaps it feels like a nice, deep massage. Or maybe it involves heat packs, stretching or exercise.

Your physician may refer you to a chiropractor or a physical therapist to help treat your aching back. Here's how these professionals work.

• **Chiropractor**

No drugs, no surgery—a chiropractor uses spinal manipulation (called "adjustments") to help relieve pressure on nerves in the back and to improve joint mobility. The chiropractor may use a deep style of adjusting or a low-force adjusting style. He may also use other procedures such as electrical stimulation (which can override the pain signals sent to your brain), massage, ultrasound (which uses sound waves to boost tissue healing) and diet changes.

An initial visit to a chiropractor will be pretty similar to a visit to your regular MD. He'll take your medical history, examine you, and maybe even study your X-rays and other lab test results. Then he'll decide on the course of treatment that will work best for you.

Chiropractic treatment plans normally run

from three to five visits per week for one to two weeks. If you're not feeling better by then, the chiropractor may try a different treatment approach or refer you to another chiropractor or a different type of health professional.

To find a chiropractor, ask your primary care physician for suggestions, ask friends and family members for the names of chiropractors they're happy with or check out *Chirodirectory.com*, which allows you to search by name, city or zip code. Remember that chiropractors must be licensed to practice in their state, and they need to have passed the National Board examinations.

• **Physical Therapist**

A physical therapist uses movement and touch to help heal a body that's in pain from arthritis, stroke, injury, diseases such as cancer and other ailments. Different types of physical therapists work with different populations (such as pediatric or geriatric) and on different disorders (such as neurological problems like spinal cord injuries). A physical therapist may use exercises, electrical stimulation, hot or cold packs, massage, ultrasound and other techniques to reduce pain and help you increase strength, flexibility and mobility.

Your physical therapist will take your health history and assess the state of your joints and muscles. From this, she'll decide on a course of treatment that may take place not just in her office, but at your home as well—meaning that she may give you exercises and stretches that you need to do on your own between visits to her office.

To find a physical therapist, ask your primary care doctor to refer you to someone he likes, and talk to your friends or family members who may have undergone physical therapy. Physical therapists have college degrees that are heavy on the sciences and postgraduate degrees in physical therapy, and they're licensed by the state in which they work.

## Giving Your Health
## Professional a Check-Up

You can get the details on the credentials and education of most physicians in the U.S. through the American Medical Association's Physician Select information at: *www.ama-assn.org/aps/amahg.htm.*

You can also check a doctor's credentials with the American Boards of her specialty and subspecialty (if she has one). For a list of boards and their contact information, visit the American Board of Medical Specialties at *www.abms.org/member.asp.* Be aware that not every health professional is board certified, as board certifications weren't commonplace more than twenty years ago. A lack of certification doesn't indicate that the health professional is not competent, only that you need to check his references another way.

Your state medical board can tell you whether a physician is currently licensed and if disciplinary action has ever been taken against her. Seek out contact information for your state medical board at the Federation of State Medical Boards: *www.fsmb.org/members.htm.*

## The Spirit Can't Be Broken

My husband Nick will never forget his trip to France: It wasn't the scenery or the history that affected him.

At the age of fifteen, adventure-seeking Nick took an exchange trip to France from his home in the UK. In Grenoble he learned the joy and the pain of mountain climbing. The joy was in conquering peaks to be master of all he surveyed. But it was a fall of about 180 feet that brought the pain.

Nick lay unconscious for ten days in a local hospital, awaking only to the sound of a Catholic priest delivering the last rites. There's nothing like being told you're dying to make you determined to live. Nick was angry. Who was this priest to decide he should die?

One of Nick's more pressing problems was an urgent call of nature. He knew few words of French and "pi-pi" wasn't one he felt able to use to a pretty nurse. He mimed elaborately the shape of a bottle.

An Algerian man who could speak a little English was fetched to act as interpreter. Convinced he knew what was needed, he dashed off and returned with a bottle of orange juice. That was good enough for Nick, who swiftly emptied the bottle before relieving himself into it.

The first his parents heard of the accident was when a whole gang of newspaper reporters turned up on their doorstep. His father had to sell his life insurance policy to pay for treatment.

The doctors treating Nick encased him in plaster from his neck to below his waist to fuse the broken bones. While he languished in a hospital far from home, his story in the French newspapers touched the hearts of some local students and they came to visit him bearing a gift of chocolate-coated cookies. Ravenous after a diet of unfamiliar food—hospital food at that—he ate the whole packet.

If there's one thing to rival the pain of a broken back it's that of a rapidly expanding stomach with nowhere to go. While he writhed in agony, a hole was cut in the plaster to accommodate it. His bulging abdomen popped out through the hole and he was able to rest easily.

Nick stayed in Grenoble Hospital for several weeks until his father arrived from the UK to escort him home. He was taken as a stretcher case to Paris where he stayed overnight at the British Military Hospital.

Nick was on three injections a day and he was

used to receiving them from a gentle nurse. Now he
was confronted by a military man of six feet-plus.
But this man's physical strength and no-nonsense
approach made for the best injection ever.

Once in the UK, Nick was treated at one of the
country's leading orthopedic hospitals, the Rowley
Bristol. He was told that treatment for his condition normally meant the spine would have to be
pinned. He would be out of the hospital in six
months, but then he would have to wear a support
belt for the rest of his life. Given the choice of this
treatment or of continuing to allow the bones to
knit naturally in plaster, which could mean two
years in the hospital, he opted for the latter.

Even in plaster Nick couldn't stay out of trouble,
and a wheelchair race with other young patients
resulted in a crash that damaged a Jaguar automobile!

Once he was able to walk, Nick got around like a
penguin. When the time came for the plaster to be
removed, it was done with great ceremony on stage
at a medical conference with people ready to catch
him if he fell. He denied them that satisfaction, but
he had to learn to walk normally again before going
on to lead a full and active life.

In his late forties Nick decided to train as a
nurse. He nearly wasn't accepted for training
because it was thought his back wouldn't be strong

enough. But he proved his fitness, rapidly rising to the top of his profession.

Now age 63, Nick is as strong and fit as many men half his age, wearing a lightweight support belt only if a heavy task demands it. He happily carries out home improvements, tends the garden and runs with the dog.

Although he remembers nothing of his accident, he can't stand heights and will cling to the arms of his chair during "cliff-hanger" scenes on television. But the one thing he has learned over the years is that a broken back needn't mean a broken life. And it certainly didn't break his spirit!

♥ *Mary Cook*

# Operation Get-Well-Soon: Surgery

Sometimes your back is giving you so much grief you just want to say, "Get me on that operating table!" After all, if a surgeon can just cut or zap your problem away, why not?

Not so fast. Surgery is a serious step, and many cases of back pain get better through less invasive methods such as physical therapy, medication, chiropractic treatment—and time. In many cases spine surgery is elective, so talk to as many medical experts as you can, do your homework and weigh your options carefully before you surge into surgery.

## Which Surgery?

If you do opt for surgery to put the kibosh on back pain, here are some of the types your physician may suggest, based on your situation:

- *Discectomy,* whether classified as *open* or *micro,* relieves pressure on the nerve roots.
- *Spinal fusion,* used for conditions like spondylolisthesis (where one vertebra slips over another one), connects vertebrae to reduce pressure on the nerve root or spinal cord.
- *Foraminotomy* is a minimally invasive procedure that widens the space around the nerves at the base of the spine.

- *Disc replacement surgery,* for people with degenerative disc disease, replaces the damaged disc with an artificial one made of metal. (This type of surgery is still experimental and performed by only a few surgeons.)
- *Spinal stenosis surgery* is for people with—you guessed it—spinal stenosis, which is a narrowing of part of the spinal canal. This surgery widens the spinal canal and is usually accompanied by spinal fusion because so much bone is removed that the spine becomes unstable and needs additional support.
- *Intradiscal Electrothermal Annuloplasty* (IDET) can help with certain types of disc herniation or degenerative disc disease. The surgeon uses a catheter to heat the affected disc to 90 degrees Celsius (194 degrees Fahrenheit) and "melt" it into a better shape.

## Before the Surgery

Before undergoing surgery, you need to prepare yourself psychologically so that you'll feel calm and confident and be ready to handle the recuperation period. Here are some actions you can take to be mentally prepared:

- *Get informed.* If you're the type of person who feels more comfortable knowing every aspect of a medical procedure (rather than the type of person who prefers to just not think about it), gather as much information as you can on the procedure and recovery from your health-care provider, the surgeon who will be performing the operation, the Internet and books. Learn what complications might arise, and make sure that you have more than one surgical opinion before agreeing to any procedure.

- *Ask for a pain control plan.* Knowing how you'll handle postoperative pain will help allay your anxiety about surgery. Ask your doctor about pain medications, ask your doctor or surgeon how much and what kind of pain you can expect, and have a number you can call (for example, for your doctor) if the pain is unexpected or gets worse.
- *Learn deep relaxation exercises.* Meditating, doing progressive relaxation (where you focus on one body part at a time) or using other relaxation techniques can help you stay calm. Ask your health-care provider for suggestions, or pick up a book like *Meditation for Dummies* (by Stephan Bodian, 2006).

## After the Surgery

Ask your doctor what you should and shouldn't do to help you recuperate quickly and successfully.

When you're recuperating, what you do (or don't do) can have an effect on how successful the surgery is. Your doctor may suggest physical therapy. The physical therapist can help you manage pain through cold packs, electrical stimulation and other means; educate you on lifestyle changes that will help you get better faster; and develop a training program that will help strengthen your body after surgery (without putting your newly operated-on back at risk). See page 82 for more on physical therapy.

## Choosing a Surgeon and a Hospital

The most important factor to consider is which surgeons and hospitals perform the most back surgeries—in general, the more experience they have, the better the outcome. Here are tips for choosing the best surgeon and hospital for you:

- Ask your doctor to suggest a surgeon to whom she would feel confident sending one of her own family members.
- Call the hospital or check out *www.qualitycheck.org* to find out if the hospital is accredited by the Joint Commission on Accreditation of Healthcare Organizations (JCAHO). Accredited hospitals have agreed to follow nationally set standards and have been evaluated by an outside body.

## What I Am Made Of

I had just come from the gear store to pick up new tent stakes for a backpacking trip I was going on next month. I turned onto Grant Avenue, driving in the right lane, when the police car in the left lane made a right-hand turn, crossing in front of my truck. I slammed on my brakes as we collided.

We both pulled over. The policeman jumped out of his car and ran to my window. "Are you okay?" he asked. "I didn't even see you. You must have been in my blind spot." He was young and panicked looking. I guessed he was a rookie.

Within minutes seven more police officers of varying rank appeared on the scene. A stranger who witnessed the accident leaned into my passenger window and urged me to talk to the rookie. Though in shock, I got out of my truck and approached the rookie. The other officers circled the rookie and then quickly and quietly escorted him into another police car and away.

The paramedics arrived and offered to take me

to the emergency room, but I declined. I was fine, I thought, no blood, no broken bones. My truck just needed a tow.

But later that night the pain started. My shoulders ached. My neck was stiff. My upper and lower back were sore. My friend and neighbor drove me first to Urgicare and then to my home in the desert.

When I woke up the next morning it hurt to move every part of my body. No matter which position I was in—lying down, sitting, standing, walking—there was no relief.

Despite my pain, I never missed work. I drove into and out of Tucson every day, an agonizing 45 minutes each way. Stabbing pain radiated across my back, into my right hip and down my leg. After work, I went to the chiropractor twice a week, to the physical therapist once. On weekends all I could do was lie on my couch. And otherwise I cried.

I was a hiker. This was who I was, how I defined myself. And now I couldn't even walk down my own unpaved street. Just walking from my truck into the house brought pain that took my breath away. My right hip had been jammed up and forward at impact as I slammed on the brakes, locking my right leg.

My whole life was structured around hiking. I lived three miles from some of my favorite trails, and commuted every day to work, so that on the weekends I could just jump out of bed and be at the trailhead within minutes.

Hiking was my sanity. It was the only time my brain quieted, after hours of placing one foot in front of the other and breathing in motion. And when I got to where I was going, I would sit and just listen, feel the rhythm of the earth pulsing through the rock where I sat, calming my own heartbeat.

Now every weekend I lay on my couch, depressed, pained and wondering who I was, now that I couldn't hike. Then I found Dave Barry's books in the library. I borrowed a stack of them, brought them home, lay in the one position that eased my back pain, and read for hours. Sometimes I laughed so hard for so long I made noises I didn't even know I could make as I struggled for air.

After weeks of this routine, I finally realized I am more than a hiker. I am more than a doer. I am me. All of me. All of my emotions, and laughter, and tears. I am all of my experiences that lead me to that moment, and all of the experiences I would have from that time forward. I am an essence that is light and sweet and exists beyond my body, beyond time, beyond pain.

Since then ten and a half years have passed. I have been in four more car accidents, all minor, each exacerbating the original injuries. I have

worked with an endless number of specialists: chiropractors, physical therapists, orthopedists, massage therapists and acupuncturists. I have changed
my diet, my posture, my gait. I have added half an
hour of prescribed exercise to every day of my life,
and still it is a rare morning I wake free of pain.
And in those ten and a half years I cannot count the
number of times I have limped off of mountains,
gritting my teeth while talking to myself as you
would to a frightened child.

But six months ago, I celebrated my fortieth
birthday by going on that long overdue backpacking trip. I went alone, and just for the night. I carried twenty-five pounds in a brand-new backpack I
had bought myself as a birthday present. I didn't go
far. But I did it. And as I walked that last stretch
back to my car, I held my hands in the air, a tri-
umphant prizefighter, and hummed the theme to
the movie *Rocky* with tears streaming down my
face. Tears of joy.

♥ *Andi Blaustein*

# Managing Medications

Pain, pain, go away. *Don't* come again another day.

If your back hurts, your health-care provider may suggest over-the-counter (OTC) or prescription drugs. He may also prescribe drugs that treat the causes of back pain—like osteoporosis—and the effects of back pain—such as depression. The different options available can be confusing, so before you pop those pills, read on to learn about the types of medications your doctor may recommend.

- **Nonsteroidal Anti-Inflammatory Drugs (NSAIDs)**

    Since inflammation can play a role in back pain, your doctor may suggest an anti-inflammatory medication such as an NSAID. Many types of NSAIDs crowd the shelves, including ibuprofin, naproxen (prescription and OTC), and COX-2 inhibitors (prescription only). Recent studies show that COX-2 inhibitors and NSAIDs may increase your risk of heart attack or stroke, so talk to your physician about your risk and possible alternatives. Some other risks of NSAIDs include stomach upset, ulcers, and liver and kidney damage (with long-term use). As always, see your doctor before starting any medication, and read and follow label instructions carefully.

## • Opioid (Narcotic) Pain Medications

Opioid medications such as codeine, hydrocodone, oxycodone and propoxyphene work by distancing you from your pain and are best used for acute and postoperative back pain. They're generally used for less than two weeks because they quickly lose their effectiveness as the body becomes used to them (a phenomenon known as *tolerance*). These drugs are strong and can become addictive, so you should take them only as prescribed and while under the care of a doctor. (In some cases, chronic back pain will be treated with long-acting opioids under close supervision by a doctor.)

## • Osteoporosis Medications

Osteoporosis medications like alendronate, risedronate, ibandronate, raloxifene, teraperatide and calcitonin use various methods to help reduce bone loss and build stronger bones. All of these drugs have the potential to cause side effects and should be taken exactly as directed by your doctor. Alendronate, residronate and ibandronate may irritate the esophagus, so you need to take them with water and avoid lying down for thirty to sixty minutes afterward. Calcitonin's only side effect is nasal irritation (it's usually prescribed as a nasal spray), but this drug is weaker than the others.

• **Muscle Relaxants**

Muscle relaxants like carisoprodol, cyclobenzaprine and diazepam work in the brain to relax the entire body, and are generally used on a short-term basis to help manage pain related to muscle spasms. Some of these drugs are habit-forming, and they may make you drowsy, so be sure to follow your doctor's instructions carefully.

• **Oral Steroids**

These are strong anti-inflammatory medications that you take for short periods of time (one to two weeks). You generally start with a high dose and taper down to a lower dose over several days. Taking oral steroids for a short period usually causes no complications— although some patients may experience shakiness, difficulty falling asleep and increased appetite—but long-term steroid use can cause weight gain, osteoporosis, stomach ulcers and other problems. People with diabetes need to be especially careful as even short-term use can make their blood sugar levels skyrocket.

### • Neuroleptic Drugs (Antiseizure Medications)

Neuroleptic drugs like gabapentin and pregabalin can be used to allay nerve pain (such as sciatica or pain from nerve degeneration). These drugs are nonaddictive and can often be taken on a long-term basis, though some patients may experience side effects like dizziness, fatigue or nausea. Be sure to follow label instructions carefully.

### • Antidepressants

Chronic back pain can cause depression, and depression can in turn make back pain worse. Your doctor may attempt to short-circuit the spiral by prescribing an antidepressant. Again, these drugs may produce side effects that you should discuss with your doctor.

## Think about . . .
### my medication history

I can show this list to my physician to help him determine the best medications for my back condition.

Medications I've taken in the past and the side effects/reactions I've experienced with them:

_____

_____

_____

_____

_____

_____

Medications I'm taking now and the side effects/reactions I've experienced with them:

_____

_____

_____

_____

_____

_____

## Child Therapist

During my first pregnancy I carried my growing baby literally on my back—or in this case on my spinal cord, causing severe pain for most of the pregnancy. After her birth the pain got worse. In fact, the pain was so unmanageable that my husband and I had to ask my mother to move in with us. Two years later I was in bed bemoaning the fact that the pain wasn't getting any better when my two-year-old came into the room to watch television with me. Out of the blue she said, "Mommy, why does your back hurt?"

What do you tell a child when she asks something like this? The truth—that during my pregnancy my back began to hurt and has only gotten worse since delivering her? Before I could even gather my thoughts together Meagan said, "If it hurts when you lie down and it hurts when you stand up, why not stand up and take me for an ice cream?"

Laughing her suggestion away, I told her to go and ask her grandmother to take her for a walk. Knowing that my mother would rather grab the ice cream carton from the freezer than walk Meagan to the store, I went back to holding my pity party for one. Finally, after watching another daytime talk show, I dozed a little and within minutes of waking up I decided, why not? Why shouldn't I get on with my life, regardless of the pain? As Meagan put it, my back was going to hurt whether I walked or lay down so I may as well do something enjoyable rather than lose my mind watching baby-daddy-mama-drama television shows.

Calling my daughter into the room, I told her to go and grab mommy's shoes because we were going walking. "Really?" she shouted as she began grabbing my legs, causing shooting pain to go straight up my spine and making me wish I could change my mind. But once you've told a child that you are going for ice cream there is no turning back.

Of course my mother thought I was crazy to walk—but then again, when didn't she have something to say about the way I was living my life? To help me out she did offer to come and get us when the pain got too bad.

Gathering our coats, we headed out the door, me hobbling and Meagan running up ahead. By the time we had gotten our ice cream my back was humming with pain and it was all I could do to stand. Luckily my daughter was absorbed in eating her ice cream cone so she didn't notice the tears of pain flowing from my eyes. I had just decided to call my mother to come pick us up when Meagan decided that she wanted to sit down. Lowering myself onto the nearest stoop, I again marveled at my daughter's uncanny ability to pick up on things. It was then that she asked me why the woman in the window was standing on her head.

Turning around, I saw that I was sitting in front of a yoga studio. *Great,* I thought, *here's another reason why I hate this pain.* I could barely walk four blocks, so the thought of taking yoga was out of the question. If it wasn't one thing it was another. Of course Meagan chose that moment to have to go potty.

Thinking quickly, I entered the yoga studio in hopes of averting an accident. I asked the receptionist if we could use their facilities. When we returned, I thanked the receptionist and mentioned that I had always wanted to join a class but with back pain and a toddler I wasn't ready. She explained to me that yoga could help with my back pain and allow me the flexibility to keep up with an active two-year-old. Within minutes, she had convinced me to not only try out a class but also enroll my daughter in the free babysitting services the studio offered.

That was four years ago. I'm now studying to become a certified yoga trainer. Meagan, who just turned seven, is still active and very precocious. My mother has since moved into an apartment nearby. I had another child two years ago and sailed through the pregnancy. I thank God every day that my daughter not only got me out of my bed but helped me see that yoga sign. There are still days that my back hurts, but they are so far and few in between that I can only believe that yoga helped me alleviate my symptoms.

*—Phenix Hall*

# Thinking Outside the Box: Complementary and Alternative Therapies

You'd think getting stuck with pins would make your back pain worse—but you'd be surprised! Alternative therapies like acupuncture, massage therapy and hypnosis are gaining mainstream acceptance in the quest to alleviate back pain.

Here are some therapies that may help you. If you choose to try one, let your health-care provider know so that he can make sure the conventional treatments he prescribes work with your alternative treatments.

• **Acupuncture**

According to traditional Chinese medicine, a life force or energy called *chi* (which we'll also see in Tai Chi and Qigong below) flows through our bodies. When the flow of *chi* is blocked, we can become ill or experience pain. Acupuncture—where a trained practitioner inserts tiny needles into certain acupuncture points on the body—can restore the flow of *chi*. (It sounds painful, but the needles are so fine that you can barely feel them.) Even if you don't believe in *chi*, you may believe that

acupuncture triggers anti-inflammatory chemicals in the body, supports the pain-killing effect
of brain chemicals called endorphins, and
boosts the immune system.

To find an acupuncturist in your area, look in
the Yellow Pages under "Acupuncture" or visit
*www.acufinder.com.* Make sure the acupuncturist
has adequate training and certification. Many (but
not all) states require acupuncture certification by
the National Certification Commission for
Acupuncture and Oriental Medicine (NCCAOM).
The NCCAOM-certified acupuncturist will have
"Dipl.Ac." after his name. Several states also have
their own exams and requirements. Visit
*www.nccaom.org* for more information.

• **Massage Therapy**
Touch can be healing; for example, babies
who aren't touched languish while those who
are touched thrive. Massage therapy, where
therapists stroke or press on certain points on
the body to relieve tension and increase the
flow of energy, has many beneficial effects: It
increases relaxation, decreases stress hormones
such as cortisol, flushes toxins from the system,
helps relieve pain and lifts the mood—and we
know that back pain is certainly a buzz-kill!

To find a massage therapist near you,

contact the American Massage Therapy Association Locator Service toll-free at 888-843-2682 or online at *www.amtamassage.org*.

• **Hypnosis**

A hypnotherapist will not swing a watch in front of your face, and he won't tell you in a fake German accent that you think you're a chicken. In reality, hypnosis works with the will, not against it. Hypnotherapists teach patients how to attain a state of openness where the subconscious mind is receptive to helpful therapeutic suggestions. Studies show that pain related to cancer, surgery, migraines and—most important for you—back injuries may respond well to hypnosis. Hypnosis can also help you with some of the conditions that make back pain worse, such as excess weight and smoking.

To find a hypnotherapist, visit the American Society of Clinical Hypnosis directory at *www.asch.net/referrals.asp#search*.

• **Yoga**

Can doing headstands help your back pain? You bet! Yoga focuses on the mind-body connection through different movements, breathing techniques and postures with names like "pigeon" and "warrior." This ancient practice can help you become more flexible, less stressed and stronger—a powerful prescription against back pain.

To find a yoga studio near you, look in your Yellow Pages under "Yoga Instruction" or visit the Yoga Centers Directory at *www.yoga-centers-directory.net.*

• **Meditation**

If your back pain is caused or made worse by stress, meditation can help. Meditation comes in many forms, and can involve repeating a *mantra* (a calming word or phrase like "peace") and focusing on the breath. Meditation isn't hard to learn, but it does take practice to reach a state of relaxation.

To learn how you can "ommm" the pain away, try a book such as *Meditation for Dummies* (by Stephan Bodian, 2006).

• **Tai Chi and Qigong (pronounced "chee gong")**

These traditional Chinese forms of exercise can relieve stress, increase stamina and strengthen balance—no more hurting your back by slipping on the ice! They consist of slow, repeated movements, breathing techniques and intense focus, which improve your body's flow of energy—that's the *chi* and *qi* in these names—to enhance your health.

To find Tai Chi instruction near you, look up "Martial Arts Instruction" or "Exercise and Physical Fitness Programs" in your Yellow Pages. For Qigong, visit the Qigong Institute at *www.qigonginstitute.org.*

## Avoiding Alternative Therapy Scams

As in all professions, alternative therapy has its share of shady products and practitioners. Follow this advice to avoid shelling out money for a bogus cure, or a therapist who cares more about his wallet than your health:

- Nix practitioners who promise a cure. A certain therapy may be able to help alleviate your pain, but no one can *guarantee* a cure.
- Avoid a practitioner who pushes you to undergo an alternative therapy that makes you feel uncomfortable.
- Beware when someone promises a treatment that uses the body's "natural cleansing ability" to heal itself.
- Avoid products (such as herbal remedies and elixirs) that supposedly have "secret ingredients."

## Avoiding Scams (cont'd)

- Pass up products that are advertised by testimonials ("'My back pain vanished instantly and my teeth are now whiter and brighter!'—Pat Z, Florida").
- Use your intuition! If something seems too good to be true, or if you have misgivings, head for the hills.

## For More Info

This is only a small selection of the alternative therapies that address pain. For the scoop on these and other therapies, visit the National Center for Complementary and Alternative Medicine at the National Institutes of Health at nccam.nih.gov, or call toll-free at 888-644-6226.

## One Newspaper at a Time

I am what I like to call a recovering foodaholic. In plain English, I am very overweight. One of the unfortunate side effects of this condition is constant back pain. Sitting, standing, lying down, carrying, lifting . . . no matter what the activity, my back is always in some state of pain.

Recently I decided to do something about this. Not only did I want to relieve the back pain that carrying around an extra 150 pounds or so creates, but I also wanted to head off all the other medical problems I knew were in my future. My biggest concern was exercise. How could I possibly move this bulk of mine around when I was already in pain? Stretching, jogging, lifting weights and all the other activities that I knew would help get the weight off just seemed impossible to do with my back always feeling like it was twisted in a knot.

So I started out slow. I got a paper route, which, to be honest, was not a weight-losing strategy at first. However, after I signed up I found out that I had to porch all of the papers. This meant that I had to get out of my car (yikes!) and physically walk the paper up the driveway and place it on the porch. This may not sound tough to many people, but to a 300-pound woman the thought of getting in and out of a car and walking up and down forty-seven driveways just didn't sound like fun. And I just knew this would aggravate my back to the point that I wouldn't be able to move at all.

Now here is where it gets interesting. Day one came and I got in and out of my car and I huffed and puffed up forty-seven driveways at two in the morning and I sweated like I hadn't done in years. I hauled myself home, got in bed and went back to sleep. When I woke up several hours later, I sat up and realized that not only was my back not throbbing in pain, as I had thought it would, but it actually felt a little bit looser.

Each week I noticed my back pain getting progressively less. Well, I figured that if just walking a little every day could help, maybe adding in a little extra exercise would help even more. I took it easy, a little at a time, doing simple exercises and other activities like playing with my children instead of popping in yet another movie for them to watch. And here came another side effect: I started to lose weight. As the weight came off, the back pain lessened.

I had always thought that I couldn't exercise because I was too large. The pain in my back, neck, legs and pretty much everywhere else, along with the sheer bulk of me, was simply too much to put through any kind of a workout routine. If I did manage to exercise, I just knew I would be in agonizing pain the next day. But just the opposite happened. This amazing human body began to function better the more I exercised. Logic had always told me that if I lost weight my back wouldn't hurt so much. After all, 300 pounds is a lot of weight for one back to carry. But the task of losing that weight just seemed too much to conquer.

So now, I'm taking baby steps. I have created a mental picture of me, newspaper carrier that I am, with 150 newspapers, each weighing a pound, strapped to my back (150 pounds being the amount I'd like to lose). Every time I lose a pound, it's like I'm throwing away one of those newspapers. Each time I toss a paper, my health is that much better, my back pain is that much less and I'm one step closer to the healthier, happier person I want to be.

I try not to look at the whole picture. I don't want to know how much I need to lose, or how much further I want to go. If I focus on the fact that I have only delivered ten papers of a 150-paper route, I'm going to want to just crawl into bed and never see the light of day again. So I don't focus on that. I take it slow. I allow myself to be proud of every moment I can sit without leaning over to crack my aching back, proud of every ounce I've lost and every ounce of mobility I've gained. And I just take each day as it comes, one newspaper at a time.

♥ *Michelle McLean*

# Ask Not What Your
# Back Can Do for You . . .

Congratulations! Your back is on its way to recovery. Keep the healing speeding along with these tips on caring for your back:

• **Kick Butts**

Smoke? Stop! Nicotine increases the risk of disc degeneration and osteoporosis (not to mention lung cancer, emphysema . . . ). Smoking even lowers your pain threshold, actually making you feel more pain! Talk to your doctor about kicking the habit; she can recommend over-the-counter or prescription medications, resources and support networks.

• **Get the Right Shoes**

Foot problems and the wrong shoes can cause back pain. If your walking or running shoes don't fit well, buy a new pair—your back is worth it. High heels throw your posture off—disaster for your back—so save the stilettos for a special occasion. If you have flat feet, if you severely overpronate (meaning the foot rolls inward when you stand or walk) or if you have Morton's toe (where the second toe is longer than the big toe), you may need corrective footwear. Visit a podiatrist for recommendations.

### • Eat Right

Excess weight (yes, even those little love handles!) can put a strain on your back. Experts say that to keep your back healthy, you should stay within ten pounds of your ideal weight. Eating right can help you shed excess pounds, and you don't have to starve yourself or follow any crazy fad diets. Ask your doctor how much you should weigh for your height, build and age, and how much you need to eat to get to or maintain that weight. Then shop for healthy, fresh, low-calorie foods like fruits, vegetables, low-fat dairy, lean meats and whole grains. Be sure to include carbs (like whole wheat bread), protein (like chicken breast) and small amounts of fat (olive oil is one of the healthier fats) in every meal, which will keep you fuller longer. Nix caloric beverages like soda for no-cal drinks like water and sugar-free iced tea.

### • Get Your Calcium

As we mention in chapter 5, calcium can help your bones stay strong. Bump up your consumption of dairy products, spinach, almonds, tofu, and calcium-fortified foods.

• **Get Moving**

Exercise strengthens the muscles that support your back, keeps you flexible, helps build bone mass and puts you on the road to slim. Talk to your doctor before starting any exercise program, and make sure your workout regimen includes cardiovascular exercise (such as biking, swimming or walking), weight training (using free weights or weight machines) and stretching. Abdominal strengthening is especially important, since your abs support your back. Remember that you can split up a single workout into several shorter sessions throughout the day if that's more convenient for you.

• **Sit Up**

Your mom was right—don't slouch! Sit up straight, especially when sitting at a desk or driving for long periods of time. Use a chair with lumbar support or get a lumbar support cushion—or, if you want to pinch pennies, just use a rolled-up towel. Using a footstool when you sit at your desk can also help.

• **Keep Your Mind Healthy**

Psychological distress such as depression and anxiety can cause back pain or make it worse. Visit your physician if you think you're depressed or overly anxious, and look into alternative treatments that can help improve your mood, such as yoga, meditation or Tai Chi (see page 107 for more details).

• **Lift Right**

We've said it before, and we'll say it again: be careful when lifting heavy objects so your back will remain healthy enough that you can haul boxes for many years to come. Bend at the knees, not at the waist, and keep the object close to your body.

## ☥ *Think about . . .*
## what I can do right now

These are the things I can do *right now* to keep
my back healthy:

___ Make an appointment with my doctor to talk
about quitting smoking.

___ Go to the bookstore or library, or go online to
research forms of exercise I'll enjoy, such as tennis, walking, martial arts, yoga or swimming.

___ Make an appointment with my doctor to ask
for help starting an exercise program.

___ Go to the grocery store and load up my cart
with fruits, veggies, whole grain breads and
pastas, low-fat dairy products, healthy oils like
olive and lean meats such as chicken breast.

___ Research gyms in my area online or through
the Yellow Pages, and visit one to ask for a
tour.

___ If my walking or running shoes are uncomfortable, go to the shoe store and ask the sales-
person to help me find a pair that fits well.

__ Create a meal plan for the week that consists of nutritious, low-calorie, filling foods.

__ Make an appointment with my physician to talk about my depression or anxiety.

__ Keep calm and relaxed with aromatherapy, a hot bath or meditation.

# Resources

Your local public library, Y, wellness center, neighborhood guild or community center are wonderful (and often free) resources for back pain-related books, periodicals, DVDs, audio- and videocassettes, massage therapy, exercise and stretching classes, as well as instruction in meditation, stress-relief, yoga, tai chi and qigong. Additionally, the following organizations and Web sites offer useful information on back ailments and back pain.

## Acupuncture

**National Certification Commission for Acupuncture and Oriental Medicine**
*http://www.nccaom.org*
Online directory of board-certified practitioners of acupuncture and Asian bodywork therapy.

**Acufinder.com**
*http://www.acufinder.com*
Online listing of over 30,000 professionals practicing acupuncture and other forms of Chinese medicine.

## Aromatherapy

**HolisticOnline.com**
*http://www.holisticonline.com/Remedies/Backpain/back_aromatherapy.htm*
This excellent online resource for alternative health treatments includes several sections devoted to back pain and offers a selection of essential oil remedies for relieving pain.

## Alternative Medicine

National Center for Complementary and Alternative Medicine (NCCAM)
*http://www.nccam.nih.gov*
NCCAM Clearinghouse
P. O. Box 7923
Gaithersburg, MD 20898
Tel: 866-644-6226
Information specialists at NCCAM's Clearinghouse can answer your questions about complementary and alternative medicine relative to back pain.

## Back Pain (General)

**MedlinePlus: Back Pain**
*http://www.nlm.nih.gov/medlineplus/backpain*
U.S. National Library of Medicine and the National Institutes of Health
8600 Rockville Pike
Bethesda, MD 20894

**Mayo Clinic.com**
*http://www.mayoclinic.com/health/back-pain*
Mayo Foundation for Medical Education and Research
Jacksonville, FL: 904-953-2000
Rochester, MN: 507-284-2511
Phoenix, AZ: 480-515-6296
Scottsdale, AZ: 480-301-8000

**American Chronic Pain Association (ACPA)**
*http://www.theacpa.org*
P. O. Box 850
Rocklin, CA 95677-0850
Tel: 800-533-3231 or 916-632-0922

**American Pain Foundation**
*http://www.painfoundation.org*
201 North Charles Street, Suite 710
Baltimore, MD 21201-4111
Tel: 888-615-PAIN (7246)

## Chiropractic

**Chirodirectory.com**
*http://www.chirodirectory.com*
National Directory of Chiropractic Headquarters
406 East 300 South, Box 305
Salt Lake City, UT 84111
Tel: 800-888-7914
Online directory of over 65,000 chiropractors.

## Massage Therapy

**American Massage Therapy Association (AMTA)**
*http://www.amtamassage.org*
500 David Street, Suite 900
Evanston, IL 60201-4695
Tel: 877-905-2700

## Qigong and Tai Chi

**The Qigong Institute**
*http://www.qigonginstitute.org*
Qigong Institute
561 Berkeley Avenue
Menlo Park, CA 94025

**Tai-Chi for Health**
*http://nccam.nih.gov/health/taichi*
National Center for Complementary and Alternative Medicine
NCCAM Clearinghouse
P. O. Box 7923
Gaithersburg, MD 20898
Tel: 866-644-6226

## Yoga

**International Yoga Centers Directory**
*http://www.yoga-centers-directory.net*
Zentrum Publishing
Box 505
Choiceland, SK, S0J 0M0, Canada
Tel: 306-428-2897

## Who Is Jack Canfield,
## Cocreator of *Chicken Soup for the Soul*®?

**Jack Canfield** is one of America's leading experts in the development of human potential and personal effectiveness. He is both a dynamic, entertaining speaker and a highly sought-after trainer. Jack has a wonderful ability to inform and inspire audiences toward increased levels of self-esteem and peak performance. He has authored or coauthored numerous books, including *Dare to Win, The Aladdin Factor, 100 Ways to Develop Student Self-Esteem and Responsibility, Heart at Work* and *The Power of Focus*. His latest book is *The Success Principles*.

*www.jackcanfield.com*

## Who Is Mark Victor Hansen,
## Cocreator of *Chicken Soup for the Soul*®?

In the area of human potential, no one is more respected than **Mark Victor Hansen**. For more than thirty years, Mark has focused solely on helping people from all walks of life reshape their personal vision of what's possible. His powerful messages of possibility, opportunity and action have created powerful change in thousands of organizations and millions of individuals worldwide. He is a prolific writer of bestselling books such as *The One Minute Millionaire, The Power of Focus, The Aladdin Factor* and *Dare to Win.*

*www.markvictorhansen.com*

## Who Is Linda Formichelli?

Linda Formichelli writes on health, wellness and other topics for *USA Weekend, Fitness, Natural Health, Women's Health* and other publications, and is a columnist for *Writer's Digest* magazine. She's the coauthor of several books, including *The Renegade Writer: A Totally Unconventional Guide to Freelance Writing Success,* which helps writers break into magazine writing and make more money by breaking the rules.

She also teaches e-courses for magazine writers. Linda lives in Concord, New Hampshire, with her writer husband and two sixteen-year-old cats. Her interests include *Archie* comics, science fiction, cats, linguistics and Thai iced tea.

*www.lindaformichelli.com.*

## Who Is Jonathan Greer, M.D.?

Dr. Jonathan Greer received his medical degree from the University of Florida. He then finished an internship and residency in internal medicine at the University of Rochester, New York. He returned to Gainesville where he completed a fellowship in Rheumatology, Immunology and Allergy. Dr. Greer has been in private practice since 1988 and currently works with the Arthritis and Rheumatology Associates of Palm Beach. Dr. Greer is also an associate clinical professor of medicine at Nova Southeastern University in Fort Lauderdale, Florida. Dr. Greer is an active lecturer to medical students, residents, practicing physicians and the lay public. His expertise focuses on the management of chronic pain, osteoporosis and musculoskeletal diseases.

## More Chicken Soup

Many of the stories in this book were submitted by readers just like you. If you would like more information on submitting a story, visit our Web site at *www.chickensoup.com*. If you do not have Web access, we can also be reached at:

Chicken Soup for the Soul®
P.O. Box 30880, Santa Barbara, CA 93130
Fax: 805-563-2945

# Contributors

**Ingrid Bairstow** is a former reporter who currently writes from her bedroom for publications in North Carolina, Virginia and Massachusetts. She found inspiration for her writing playing with and caring for her children and following her Marine Corps husband around the country (or waiting for him to return from Iraq).

**Janice Bazen** is a registered nurse with Interim Home Health. She began writing as a hobby in 2001. When Janice is not working, she enjoys camping, reading, fishing and following the NASCAR series. Janice was previously published in *Chicken Soup for the NASCAR Soul*.

**Andi Blaustein** is an adult educator living and working in Colorado. She recently successfully completed a three-day backpack trip in Paria Canyon on the Utah-Arizona border—a trip she has dreamed about taking for more than ten years.

**Mary Cook** is a U.K.-based freelance writer and former newspaper reporter. Her articles, short stories and poems have appeared in numerous publications, both in print and online. A Nichiren Shoshu Buddhist, she lives in the rural county of Lincolnshire with her husband, Nick, their Border terrier, Brucie, and cat, Lotus.

**Phenix Hall** lives and works in New York City. Her passions include volunteering for local soup kitchens, reading and enjoying the outdoors. Phenix currently freelance writes for several local publications and has dreams of one day becoming a published book author.

**Phyllis Hanlon** freelances from her home in central Massachusetts. She has written hundreds of articles for several different publications, including *America*, *Bride & Groom*, *Massage Magazine*, *Road King*, *St. Anthony Messenger*, *Skin Deep* and others. And she always finds time to get a massage.

**Hilary Hart** is a freelance writer who teaches writing and literature at the University of Oregon.

**Amanda Kendle** is a wandering Australian who has lived in various parts of Europe and Asia. Traveling, writing and understanding different people and cultures are her greatest passions. You can learn more at *www. amandakendle.net*.

**Michelle McLean** is a twenty-nine-year-old mother of two. Michelle has a B.S. in history, and will soon begin work on her Master's. An avid writer, she does freelance work, and is working on getting some children's stories and her first novel published.

**Darcy Silvers** is a native Floridian who now calls the Philadelphia area her home. A freelance writer, her career has spanned the gamut from journalism to advertising, marketing and public relations. When she's not nursing her aching back, she's busy volunteering, dancing and looking for new story ideas. Contact her at *http://home.comcast.net/~thehiredhand/*.

**Dr. Paul Wright** is the Department Chair of Physical Education & Recreation Administration at Southern Virginia University in Buena Vista, Virginia. Dr. Wright is also the collegiate coach of track and cross-country. His teams have won ten USCAA National Small School titles in the last five years.

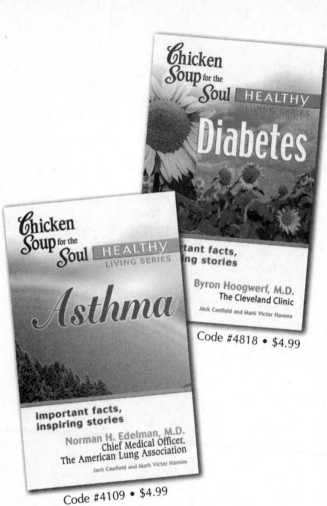

Code #4818 • $4.99

Code #4109 • $4.99

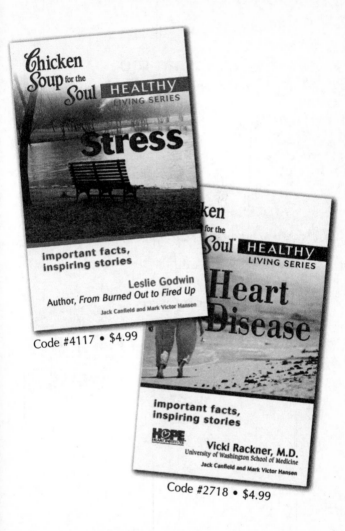

Code #4117 • $4.99

Code #2718 • $4.99

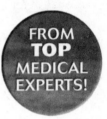